PORTAL TO HEAVEN

Opening up your Magic with Womb Healing
A Womb Healing Workbook from
the Sacred Rose Order

JULIE WILSON

DEDICATION

To my mom for bringing so much to my awareness in my teenage years and sending me to that first healing session that started my journey back to me.

I love you.

A very special thank you goes to my daughter, Megan. She continues to amaze me daily. She has taught me unconditional love on a level I didn't know existed. She is my inspiration, my catalyst, and the fire that pushes me to be the best version of myself. She is the reason this book came to life. There are no words for the gratitude I have for her and how much she has helped my heart heal.

DEDICATION

TABLE OF CONTENTS

INTRODUCTION

Hi, lovely reader! My name is Julie Wilson, and I'm writing this workbook to share many of the tools, practices, and information that have helped me in my healing journey. I sometimes felt like a fish out of water when I started working on myself. I stumbled my way through what felt like a very confusing process at times. This workbook highlights the things that helped me most in an order that I felt would be easiest from start to finish. There are many links to videos and exercises, so you will have both visual and written text to go on. But first, let me tell you about me.

Let's go back to the beginning. My younger years were filled with imaginary friends and dancing around the house with a broom. When I got home from school, I always made a beeline to my cassette player and turned on my music. My mom made whole-made bread and my absolute favorite chicken and dumplings (always from scratch). She had an old ringer washer, and the laundry was always hanging outside, blowing in the wind. It smelled so good, and I still smile when I do laundry, remembering my younger years. I would run between the hanging sheets, hide in her Cannas that were taller than me, might I add, and play with my outside cats. (I was an animal lover; we had 16 cats at one time). The landlord's horses could be seen from my bedroom window in a strange little house with no bedroom doors and a big pot belly stove. I had many nights of blanket rides on a sheet through the square doorways. I loved scary movies and throwing spaghetti at the wall to see if it was done.

The memories were good. One day, my dad caught the toaster on fire, putting a slice of whole made bread in. My mom said it needed a trim, but he stuck it in anyway, then ran outside with the toaster and the flames coming out the top. I still laugh to this day at the image of him running out of the house like a cartoon character as fast as he could. I was content and happy playing by day and watching the stars with my dad by night. He used to say I'll be up there one day; just look up. The big dipper was always what we looked for. He also always told me to follow my heart.

My parent's divorce at age 5 left me having to choose a parent to live with, so I stayed with my dad. I was a normal kid trying to navigate parents splitting up. Things went along okay for a while.

I had those key, fabulous moments. The day I learned how to ride a bike was magical. I could feel the wind in my hair and felt so free. (It was the 80s, and kids just played outside and came in when it got dark.) I tell my daughter all the time I wish we could timewarp back to my childhood era sometimes so she could go ride around the subdivision without being watched. But we live in different times now. Back to it, we were the only house on the street, so I could pretty much ride back and forth for hours—my banana seat and pedaling as fast as I could. My hair would be impossible to brush when I went in. So day after day, I would swear to myself I wasn't riding that stupid bike again because my hair was so tangly. But we all know what happened the next day and the next and the next.

Then things started to change. My dad changed. He seemed sad all the time. I suddenly started questioning what was wrong and what was going on. Then it got even stranger. I began to lose time. It was like I went to bed and woke up, but the hours were just gone. The potbelly stove was hot one minute and cold the next, and I couldn't understand where the time went. I still remember standing there perplexed, thinking I must be losing my mind at the young age of 7.

One night, I remembered why time was missing and some of

the sexual abuse, so I asked my mom if I could come live with her. Many of my memories of the abuse were still left blocked, so I just went on about my childhood and went to live with my mom in an apartment on my grandparent's farm. I was raised around homegrown vegetables, driving trucks in the field when I could barely touch the gas pedal (my favorite!), throwing cantaloupes and sometimes watching them all fall as I hit the brakes too hard, and eating watermelon off the tailgate.

Every spring, the flower planting began. My grandparents also had a huge glass greenhouse; I absolutely loved it in there. I would skip down the long rows, taking in all the beauty and scents of all the different flowers. I also loved playing store with my grandma and would take another purse home each day from the pile for sale. My mom told me later there were hundreds she had unloaded from the attic. I never processed what happened with my dad. I gained a ton of weight during fourth grade that didn't come off until high school (with the help of an eating disorder), and I didn't really fit in with anyone. The next few years were kind of a blur.

At the age of 16, I read a book called The Mists of Avalon and was immediately lost in it. I read the whole book in a matter of a few days. My priestess memories began returning, although I didn't quite understand them. I just thought I really liked the book.

My mom started reading self-help books like Chicken Soup for the Soul and learning about Buddhism. Because she got into this stuff, it led me to see alternative paths and opened me up to different ways of thinking. I started listening to classical music, meditating, and chanting. I found Pachelbel's Cannon in D with Ocean Waves on CD (CDs were then the trend, and the music store was my favorite place to go).

I don't remember the name of the chanting CD, but I remember going to the void. That place where there is just nothing and time ceases to exist. When I came back to my body, I was startled and said out loud, "I'm not ready." I tried for years to figure out what that even meant; I wasn't ready for what? I kept asking, but there was no answer. I shut my spiritual gifts down and went on with my life.

My father's death from a heart attack sent me spiraling at age 17. My mom was in Germany when I found him, which made it even worse as she was inaccessible for a good 24 hours until she got home. I just knew something was wrong and had to go see him that night. It was a bit of another blur for the next few years. His death opened up all that had been pushed down and sealed away and sent me on a wild journey, leading to a fake ID and a bit of chasing highs with party scenes. While I wouldn't suggest this route, it had its place in my story, and I found freedom from what I was carrying at the time. I was luckily always protected and safe in the spaces and friends I found.

I was still functioning but looking to numb the pain and codependent guilt I carried. I felt shame and responsibility for moving out and leaving my dad alone when I was a child, even though I couldn't stay in that house for another minute. I rebottled my pain, emotions, and everything I couldn't understand about what had happened until much later in my life.

Fast forward to college and climbing the corporate ladder. I got my act together and managed to get an Associate Degree in Accounting and later went on to get a Bachelor's in Business. I thought I was on my way to living the American Dream.

Dating was interesting as I still had much to learn and heal. I found my soulmate after a few relationships and a bit more confidence in who I was, and I knew I would marry him as soon as our eyes locked. I didn't know how I knew (I still had my gifts somewhat shut down), but nevertheless, I knew. It is still my favorite story to tell my daughter. This feeling just came over me when I was around him. He felt safe and fun. It was like those childhood dreams you think you'll feel when you fall in love.

In 2009, I was in a car accident where the driver behind me sneezed, hit me, and spun my car up an embankment. It was the morning of my wedding day, and something happened as I stood there by my undrivable car. I knew nothing would stop me from marrying my husband. There was this connection to my higher self that I hadn't felt since my teenage years came back over me. I said, "I'm ready," though still not sure ready for what, but never the less ready for something. My mind went back to that 16-year-old me and thought well, now that I'm ready, I guess we will see what that means.

Later, I would understand this was the reopening of the gifts I had shut down. I was ready to understand the unseen world and the quantum field. I was tired of questioning and prepared to dive head-first into the abyss of the unknown. But I am getting ahead of myself. My physical body was the priority as the pain soon set in from the wreck. I suffered a neck injury that took years to heal. I was forced to be still, not something I did well back then, but the beginning of the surrender was upon me.

Next up was the pregnancy journey. I was destined to be a mom; it was just something I felt in every part of my body and soul. However, I also knew deep down that it wouldn't be easy. I happily went off birth control as it was making me nauseous by the time I stopped taking it. So, the red flags started signaling. That's when my body started screaming at me. Ovarian cysts that were so bad I thought it had to be my appendix one night at dinner. It was not, and that was when I really started wondering what the heck was going on. Then the back pain followed (endometriosis). A few years passed, and still no pregnancy.

The process was long. The doctors wanted to do expensive fertility treatments as they couldn't find what was wrong. I knew I needed surgery from my research and intuitive nudge that pinged this was the only way. Imagine going in and saying my intuition is guiding me a certain way. Can we bypass what you suggest and just go with it? I assumed I would have been met with laughter. But by the third doctor, I walked in and told her I felt the surgery to remove the endometriosis was the only way. She not only listened but agreed. The entire process of finding a doctor who would listen had taken a toll on my emotional body, but I was finally heard. I felt relief, but it was short-lived as that surgery led to more frustration and anger at how temporary the relief was.

This was by far the most physically painful part of my journey between cysts, endometriosis, and my neck injury. There were many sleepless nights and tears along the way, followed by anxiety—the classic sign of an unregulated nervous system.

I wasn't yet aware of just how powerful we are or what unhealed trauma does to the physical body, so it was the fastest route to pregnancy at that time. I stopped wondering how I knew and just went with what my higher self was trying to tell me. The needed surrendering began to deepen, followed by the inner child work. Without knowing it, the healing process in my womb had begun.

I had many a breakdown before getting to where I am today. One day, my husband even told me he would get me as many dogs as I wanted if I couldn't get pregnant. I started laughing as the image of a house full of dogs hit my mind. I asked him if he knew what he had just agreed to. His reply was simply an 'Oh boy'. We went and got a second puppy shortly after.

I had a small window to try and get pregnant, as that surgery wasn't a permanent fix. The day I took the pregnancy test, I knew before I even saw the results. I knew she was a girl, but I didn't tell anyone until I got the blood test back. Somewhere in my mind, I was terrified if I said it out loud too fast, I would jinx it. I wanted concrete proof. So, my long-awaited pregnancy was finally here. For those nine months, I was focused on her.

Still, I was frustrated, confused, and unsure of what was causing all the problems. I wanted answers as to why my body was in so much pain. Where was the underlying issue? How was it so hard to get pregnant when I saw others pregnant within a month or two? What had I done wrong? The questions started stacking up.

With the birth of my daughter in 2013, my body was having even more trouble. I started doing yoga, meditating, and listening to every podcast I could find about how to heal the body. What my mom had exposed me to during my teens kicked back in, and I wanted to understand what was going on from more than a medical diagnosis. I couldn't believe she was actually here—this beautiful little angel. There were nights I walked for hours up and down the hall so she would sleep. I loved nurturing her little soul and listening to her sleep on my shoulder when too many teeth were coming in at once.

In 2017, I received my first shamanic reiki energy healing session, and I knew I wanted to learn everything I could about energy work. I was a wreck between an unregulated nervous system and anxiety bordering on panic attacks. My mom, not knowing what to do to help, asked if I would want to do an energy healing session she found at a local healing center. I had tarot readings before and was super open to energy work, but I didn't know much about it. At the end of that session, I was taken back to pure childhood joy with an image of me as a child running through the grass and laughing. I had to know more about this work.

First, I started with yoga teacher training; however, I never finished certification from an overextended knee, which I was slow to recover from. Reiki was next (I no longer do this, but it was the first spiritual course I finished). Then, the Akashic records, DNA Activation, Quantum healing, Auric field work,

Light language, Timeline healing and clearing, Ancestral healing, more minor certifications, and some long-term six-month mentorship programs to expand my gifts.

Many womb healing courses or programs don't simply, practically, and foundationally lay out the tools and processes to heal the womb. This work is crucial to diving further into the priestess path and Rose lineage work. The basics of healing must first be understood. This includes working with your body and connecting with your higher self. I took Womb Healing courses, where the main focus was to listen to meditations and connect with the energy of the Rose Orders, but I felt like I was missing something. While I resonate deeply with priestess work, it wasn't what was needed initially.

I just needed good old tools, steps, understanding, and enough options to find my flow. If you are called to work with the Rose lineages, you will know as your healing journey progresses, you will naturally begin to remember your past lives working with these energies. Healing brings access to new levels of consciousness, which will naturally bring in the ability to unlock more information and guide you to the next step.

Fast forward to the present day, with the retrieval of memories, multidimensional aspects, and so much self-worth, I honestly didn't think it was possible to be this happy. The path to happiness is not always easy, but it is always worth it. I realized just how much was related to the womb. Healing takes accountability and determination, but the journey doesn't have to be as hard as I made it. We can use the tools to learn to ebb and flow, not attach to what comes through us, and bounce back to inner child bliss in the blink of an eye (ok, well, some shifts take a bit longer, but you get what I mean).

The womb is the second heart. It is where souls are born (a magical portal and the only natural way to bring human life into this world!), hence where the title of the book came from.

Healing the womb can release emotional blocks connected to many things. It plays a significant role in controlling your destiny. It helps you express your wants and needs freely and realize your potential. But most importantly, it enables you to open up to more life-force energy for mental, emotional, spiritual, and physical well-being.

The download to create this workbook is something I hold very dear to my heart and my soul. My work as a priestess of the Sacred Rose carried me when times got rough and helped me work through the layers, as I hope this workbook is a road map for many others to begin to take back their joy and happiness. We will journey into all the places ready to heal.

And this is where we will begin our womb healing journey - in understanding and knowledge with the tools to heal...

PORTAL TO HEAVEN

Opening up Your Magic with Womb Healing
A Womb Healing Workbook from
the Sacred Rose Order

This QR Code has all the links in this book in order as you go.

If there is ever an issue with this QR code, email healingwithjw@gmail.com for a list of links.

CHAPTER 1
EXPLANATION OF WOMB HEALING

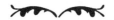

Womb healing holistically addresses emotional, physical, or spiritual imbalances that may exist within the womb space or reproductive system.

Womb healing often addresses fertility, menstruation, and childbirth issues. However, it can also be a powerful tool for healing emotional trauma, such as past sexual abuse, unhealthy partners, or other forms of trauma that may be stored in the body.

The womb, or the uterus, is a powerful organ in a woman's body that can create and nurture life. It is the second heart and a powerful portal that brings souls into this world. However, the womb can also be a site of trauma from many life experiences, such as miscarriage, childbirth, medical procedures, or sexual abuse. There are many times emotional and spiritual healing needed when physical traumas happen.

Womb healing involves exploring and addressing any past traumas or imbalances that may be affecting the health and well-being of the womb, as well as developing practices and habits to support the overall health of the womb. Using practices such as meditation, yoga, breathwork, quantum healing, connecting with the Divine Feminine, and taking herbs and supplements can support physical healing.

Womb healing is important not only for physical health but also for emotional and spiritual well-being. By addressing traumas or imbalances in the womb, individuals can experience better emotional stability, physical health, and a deeper connection to their feminine energy.

WHY IS THE WOMB CALLED A PORTAL?

The womb has been described as a portal because it is the gateway through which new life enters this physical world. It is also a portal because it is a powerful, energetic center intimately connected to the body, mind, and spirit.

In many spiritual traditions, the womb is considered a sacred space with the potential for creation and transformation. In some cultures, the womb is the source of a woman's intuitive wisdom and spiritual power.

The idea of the womb as a portal in the context of shamanic practices is believed to be a gateway to other realms of consciousness. In these traditions, the womb is a channel through which a person can connect with the spiritual world and receive guidance and healing. By honoring and nurturing the womb, we can tap into our creative power and connect with the sacred dimensions of life.

BENEFITS OF WOMB HEALING

There are many potential benefits to womb healing, including:

Physical healing: Trauma or imbalances in the womb can impact reproductive health and contribute to issues such as menstrual pain, fertility problems, and complications during pregnancy and childbirth. Addressing any physical trauma or imbalances in the womb can help improve reproductive health, reduce menstrual pain and discomfort, and support overall physical health.

Emotional healing: Issues in the womb can impact emotional well-being, and addressing these issues can help individuals feel more grounded, emotionally stable, and connected to their feminine energy. It can also lead to less anxiety, depression, and overall difficulty with intimacy and relationships.

Spiritual growth: The womb is often seen as a sacred space in many spiritual traditions, and connecting with and healing this space can lead to a deeper sense of spiritual connection (not only to spiritual gifts but to source as well) and growth.

Increased creativity: The womb is often associated with creativity and creation, and by healing and nurturing this space, individuals may experience a greater sense of creative inspiration and expression.

Empowerment: Addressing past trauma in the womb can be a powerful act of self-care and empowerment, helping individuals take control of their physical, emotional, and spiritual health.

Breaking cycles of trauma: Looking at and healing past trauma in the womb can help break cycles of trauma and support future generations in healthier relationships with their bodies and reproductive health.

Improved relationships: Examining past traumas or imbalances in the womb can lead to greater emotional stability and a more profound sense of self-awareness, which can improve relationships with others.

Overall, womb healing can be a transformative and empowering process that supports physical, emotional, and spiritual well-being to help women connect with their feminine energy and personal power. Addressing womb trauma is vital for individual and generational well-being; we heal the lineage in both directions when we heal our wombs.

CHAPTER 2

UNDERSTANDING THE WOMB

ROLE OF THE WOMB IN THE REPRODUCTIVE SYSTEM

The uterus (womb) is the organ in the female body where a fertilized egg implants and develops into a fetus during pregnancy. There are times when medical intervention is needed. In my situation, surgery was necessary for endometriosis to get pregnant. My real issues started with ovarian cysts and severe pain during periods. The back pain and endometriosis followed, then anxiety to top it off. I later healed my physical problems with many of the tools in this book and am now symptom-free, but intuitively, following those first nudges led me to surgery.

When my back pain returned within weeks after the birth of my child, I wanted a better solution and began learning everything I could about energy work and healing the body. I tried medication for the anxiety, but nothing worked long-term, and the side effects led me to even more issues. As I stepped more into my power, I began to unpack the trauma that was causing the physical pain. I learned firsthand how important healing the womb and the body is.

Infertility is one of the most heart-wrenching journeys I have ever had to experience, and I didn't understand how everything was linked. Our minds are powerful things, and the suppression of my childhood memories of sexual abuse kept me safe until I was ready to understand what had fully happened. Although my mind was safe, my body was another story.

Living year after year with an unregulated nervous system caused physical damage as my body sent alarms, wanting me to notice something wrong. I never really left fight or flight, or should I say freeze, which is where I was. It was a long process and, as I look back, frustrating in ways because I just wanted answers. I was willing to do the work, whatever that looked like, but I didn't know what to do. I just needed someone to explain the process and the tools and remind me to have more fun. *We don't know what we don't know until we do.* So, regret is not something I focus on for long. I keep it moving because it keeps improving, and every time I tell myself I can't believe this is my life, something even more spectacular happens. If this shaves off some uncertainty and adds hope to other women on their journeys, I am happy to share what got me here.

Then there is the lineage piece after we heal ourselves. I questioned if a person could do these acts of abuse to children; what did that mean for history repeating itself if I didn't dig deeper into healing the lineage? Sexual abuse as a child changes how you parent your children. I didn't want my daughter to carry the burden forward of the trauma I held. Since the mother-child relationship in the womb is so intimate, as well as the fact my C-section was traumatic, that mama bear, warrior, protective energy came up. Once ignited my mission became more about protecting all the children and their energy. Many of us came here to be the cycle breakers. If you are reading this book, I would bet you are here to do just that.

SPIRITUAL AND ENERGETIC SIGNIFICANCE OF THE WOMB

The womb is considered to have significant spiritual and energetic importance in many cultures and spiritual traditions worldwide. In some belief systems, the womb is seen as the source of creation, the seat of the Divine Feminine, and a powerful center of feminine energy. In many ancient cultures, the womb was revered as a sacred space due to its significance as the only natural way to bring human souls into this world.

In addition to its physical functions, the womb is believed to hold emotion and energetic imprints from past experiences, including trauma, grief, and joy. (We will go through many ways to release negative experiences later in this work.)

Many spiritual practices also emphasize connecting with the womb through meditation, visualization, and energy work. By connecting with the womb, women can tap into their feminine power and intuition and access a more profound sense of creativity and spiritual connection.

There are seven main chakras associated with our physical bodies. Meditation and the chakra system are where I started to understand us as energy beings. The sacral or second chakra is related to the womb.

Healing the womb can release emotional blocks connected to many things. It plays a significant role in controlling your destiny. It helps you express your wants and needs freely. Help us realize our potential and open up to more life-force energy for mental, emotional, spiritual, and physical well-being.

The sacral chakra, also known as the womb chakra, is the home to your emotions, creative energy, power center, development for babies, business, projects, life-force energy, and primal sexual force. It is directly connected to your root chakra, the safety center.

Here are some Sacral Chakra lessons we deal with in this lifetime: codependency, independence, apathy, overeating, storing old emotions, taking on others' energy as your own, and learning to decipher your and another's feelings.

These lessons and blocks (also known as trauma or wounds) can cause a plethora of issues, and those issues leak out into your relationship with money, with your children, with all those around you, and your relationship with yourself, including self-worth. It touches literally every aspect of your life. This is where we can absorb the feelings of others, judge the self and relationships, and clear self-destructive patterns and behaviors.

Overall, the womb is a powerful center of feminine energy, representing the power of creation, intuition, and profound impact, and is viewed as a sacred space. Practices that honor connecting with the womb can bring healing, balance, and spiritual growth.

CHAPTER 3
WOMB TRAUMA

TYPES OF WOMB TRAUMA

Womb trauma can refer to a range of experiences that negatively impact the womb's physical, emotional, and energetic well-being. Some examples of types of womb trauma include:

Sexual abuse: Sexual abuse can profoundly impact the health and well-being of the womb. It can lead to physical damage, relationship issues, and emotional trauma, manifesting as tension, pain, or discomfort in the pelvic region.

Medical trauma: Medical procedures, such as surgeries, abortions, or childbirth complications, can also lead to trauma in the womb. Even pap smears can be traumatic. These experiences can cause physical damage and emotional distress, leading to pelvic pain, endometriosis, or post-traumatic stress disorder (PTSD).

Miscarriage or stillbirth: Experiencing the loss of a pregnancy through miscarriage or stillbirth can also cause trauma in the womb. This can lead to physical symptoms such as pain or discomfort and emotional trauma such as grief, depression, or anxiety.

Infertility: Struggling with infertility or undergoing fertility treatments can also cause trauma in the womb. This can lead to physical symptoms such as pain or discomfort and emotional distress such as anxiety, depression, or feelings of inadequacy and unworthiness.

Cultural and ancestral trauma: Trauma can be passed down through generations, including trauma related to cultural or ancestral experiences. This can manifest as physical symptoms or emotional distress related to the womb, such as chronic pelvic pain or difficulty conceiving.

Overall, womb trauma can have a range of causes and effects and may require different approaches to healing and recovery depending on the individual's experiences and needs.

SIGNS AND SYMPTOMS OF WOMB TRAUMA

Womb trauma can significantly impact an individual's physical, emotional, and spiritual well-being. Here are some examples:

Physical health: Womb trauma can lead to various physical health issues, including chronic pelvic pain, menstrual irregularities, weight gain, infertility, and sexual dysfunction. Trauma can also increase the risk of developing endometriosis, fibroids, or pelvic inflammatory disease.

Pelvic pain or discomfort: Womb trauma can cause physical pain or discomfort in the pelvic region, including the uterus, ovaries, or fallopian tubes.

Menstrual irregularities: Trauma in the womb can also affect menstrual cycles, generating irregular periods, heavy bleeding, or painful cramping.

Sexual dysfunction: Trauma can also affect sexual function and pleasure, leading to difficulty with arousal, pain during intercourse, or other sexual dysfunctions.

Fertility issues: Trauma can also affect fertility, making it difficult to conceive or carry a pregnancy to term.

Chronic health issues: Trauma in the womb can also contribute to chronic health issues such as endometriosis, fibroids, or pelvic inflammatory disease.

Emotional well-being: Womb trauma can also have a profound impact on emotional well-being, producing feelings of anxiety, depression, or post-traumatic stress disorder (PTSD). Trauma can also affect self-esteem, confidence, and feelings of safety and security.

Emotional distress: Trauma in the womb can also cause emotional distress, such as anxiety, depression, or post-traumatic stress disorder (PTSD).

Spiritual well-being: Trauma in the womb can also impact spiritual well-being, causing a sense of disconnection from one's body or the Divine Feminine. This can lead to feelings of disempowerment, lack of creativity, and difficulty accessing intuition or other spiritual gifts.

Energetic imbalances: Trauma in the womb can also cause energetic imbalances, showing up as feelings of disconnection, loss of creativity, or a sense of disempowerment.

Interpersonal relationships: Trauma can also impact interpersonal relationships, contributing to intimacy, trust, and communication difficulty. Trauma can also affect one's ability to form healthy attachments or maintain healthy boundaries.

Womb trauma can significantly impact a woman's overall health and well-being and may require a comprehensive approach to healing and recovery that addresses physical, emotional, and spiritual needs.

CHAPTER 4
THE 21-DAY ROADMAP

Before we get into the healing sections, I wanted to share a 21-day roadmap to get started. It takes 21 days to anchor in a new habit. The practices in this 21-day road map are many of the things listed in this workbook, but this was a quick reference to get an idea of what daily planning could look like. If you are new to doing this work, I want it to be easy and natural so you can find your flow and have small, manageable daily steps. (*The video links can be found in the QR code in order as they go in the book.*)

Please take a moment and paint, draw, or color a picture of yourself. It can just be colors or lines, symbols, etc. It is more about the feeling, the energy, and not the actual image. The goal is to ignite the sacral energy and create a starting point for this healing journey. When the 21 days are over, you will draw and compare a new image. (You can paint and play with your artistic expression as much as you like; in fact, I highly suggest getting in touch with your creative side.)

Print this form* 21 times and do it daily. The same word will be written in each blank slot. I did not create this form (Jason Estes from MTVO.org created this, but I did this a few years ago and found it very healing around my money stories). For the focus of this workbook, please use a word or phrase that focuses on your womb healing journey. A few suggestions would be grief, suffering, trauma, pain, delusion, misunderstandings, fear, attachments, and unprocessed energies. You can also do more

---

* Source: *https://www.facebook.com/MTVOTeam/posts/2587305374815798*

than one at a time, but if you miss a day, you have to start over on day one.

https://img1.wsimg.com/blobby/go/3bc5adb9-12c6-470c-9266-c38fdefe5382/Light%20of%20God%20Sheet.pdf

DAY 1

1. Higher self-meditation *https://youtu.be/Vo9vGFbzYEg*
2. Gratitude Practice (make a list of what you are grateful for)
3. Nervous System reset https://www.youtube.com/watch?v=dKBEqL4PZvQ
4. Journal Prompt: What does my womb want to tell me?

DAY 2

1. Inner Child Meditation https://youtu.be/ZNci8FjBKk0?si=jPHylKCoiD5cERig
2. Eat fruit and veggies or make a smoothie.
3. Dance for at least five minutes and paint or draw an image from your soul
4. Journal Prompt: What does my inner child crave that she has not received?

DAY 3

1. Sacred Flame Healing and Yoni Mudra <u>https://youtu.be/Ib3m4MEOmGQ?si=pGUHOETwQVQEyV43</u>

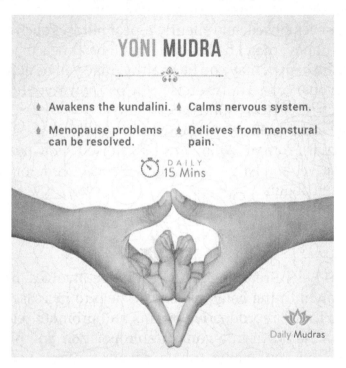

2. Womb Yoga <u>https://youtu.be/hw8UjuXDcFU</u>
3. Hot salt bath or sauna
4. Journal Prompt: Where has holding onto pain, discomfort, trauma, or stagnant energy hurt me?

DAY 4

1. Higher Timeline meditation *https://youtu.be/HZaL42XR0yQ?si=QzKRDvIXGCLEyaFI*
2. Ho'oponopono <u>https://youtu.be/2TePAocURL</u>
3. Chant OM
4. Journal Prompt: Where do I blame myself or others for things in the past?

DAY 5

1. Loving-Kindness Meditation: This technique involves cultivating love, kindness, and compassion towards yourself and others. Sit in a comfortable position with your eyes closed, and silently repeat phrases such as "May I be happy, may I be healthy, may I be at peace" or "May you be happy, may you be healthy, may you be at peace."
2. Nervous system exercise https://www.youtube.com/watch?v=L1HCG3BGK8I&t=2s
3. Physical exercise 5-15 minutes
4. Journal Prompt: When I talk to myself, is it positive or negative, and why or what do I criticize and am hard on myself about?

DAY 6

1. Deep Belly Breathing: This technique involves breathing deeply into the belly, which can help to increase oxygen flow to the reproductive organs and promote relaxation. Sit or lie down in a comfortable position and place one hand on your belly. Inhale deeply through your nose, allowing your belly to expand, and exhale fully through your mouth, allowing your belly to contract.
2. Walking Meditation: This technique involves bringing your attention to the physical sensations of walking, such as the movement of your feet and the feeling of the ground beneath you. Walk slowly and deliberately, focusing on your body and surroundings.
3. Eat something Earthy that will ground your energy, such as carrots, pumpkin, turnips, potatoes, turmeric, ginger, or sweet potatoes.
4. Journal Prompt: Where in my body do I feel pain or discomfort when connecting with my womb space?

DAY 7

1. Womb Activation Meditation https://youtu.be/5JHDDFlKINk?si=FIBBzvliE7jPG7u1
2. Ujjayi Breath: This technique is also known as "ocean breath" and involves breathing deeply through the nose while constricting the back of the throat. This can help to regulate the breath and promote relaxation. Sit or stand comfortably, inhale deeply through your nose while constricting the back of your throat. Exhale entirely through your nose, tightening the back of your throat.
3. Body Scan Meditation: This technique involves bringing your attention to different body parts, one at a time, and noticing any sensations or tension you may be holding. Lie down in a comfortable position, close your eyes, and bring your attention to your toes. Move your attention slowly up your body, noticing each part until you have released any tension.
4. Journal Prompt: What is the best way to heal and repair the trauma inside my body?

DAY 8

1. Guided Imagery: This technique can help to reduce stress and promote relaxation. Sit or lie comfortably, and imagine a healing light or energy surrounding your womb. Visualize this healing energy filling your body and bringing balance and harmony to your reproductive system.
2. Artistic Expression: Engaging in creative activities such as drawing, painting, or dancing can help release emotions and allow self-expression.
3. Shaolin Qigpng 15-Minute Daily Routine https://youtu.be/y2RAEnWreoE
4. Journal Prompt: Where do you feel unsafe, unseen, or unheard?

DAY 9

1. Decree to Clear Energy (say out loud)

    I do not consent to any form of tech, negative energy, or manipulation that will feed on my weaknesses and undermine my authority to be sovereign and in my personal power.

    I do not consent to any form of negative interference with my energy. I am supported by and connected to pure higher dimensional frequencies, and all impurities are continuously cleared and removed, whether from conscious or unconscious agreement and understanding.

    I am supported and protected by my internal guidance and higher self-connection. I go through the channel of my soul signature to receive messages or guidance, ensuring I am keeping my channel clear and clean.

    I return to my centered state of existence with grace and ease whenever I feel unbalanced, or my energy is low.

    Upgrades can be adjusted to fit my speed of integration at any time by simply checking in with my body and what is needed.

    I replace all that no longer serves my highest good with the best intentions for growth and prosperity in all timelines across all planes of reality.

2. Somatic Exercise: see where you may have used these coping mechanisms and how to journal about how you would have liked to have handled the situation differently.

    The "fit in" response involves trying to blend in with the crowd or conform to the expectations of others to avoid being noticed or singled out. This response is often seen in social situations, where an individual may feel pressure to conform to the norms and expectations of a group to avoid rejection or criticism.

The "fawn" response involves trying to please others or appease a perceived threat to avoid harm. This response is often seen in individuals who have experienced trauma or abuse and may include strategies such as people-pleasing, apologizing excessively, or avoiding conflict at all costs.

The "fight or flight" response involves confronting or attempting to escape the perceived threat. This response is often seen in situations with a clear and immediate danger, such as a physical altercation or a natural disaster.

The "freeze" response involves becoming immobilized or "stuck" in the face of a perceived threat. This response is often seen when an individual feels overwhelmed or helpless and may include a sense of dissociation or detachment from the situation.

3. Somatic exercises for difficult emotions https://youtube. com/shorts/ivToyrWC9bs?feature=share
4. Journal Prompt: What is the best way to move stagnant energy to allow more light into the areas needing light?

DAY 10

1. Alternate Nostril Breathing: This technique involves breathing through one nostril at a time, which can help balance the body's energy flow. Sit comfortably, and use your right thumb to close your right nostril. Inhale deeply through your left nostril, and then use your right ring finger to close your left nostril. Exhale entirely through your right nostril, and then inhale deeply through your right nostril. Close your right nostril with your thumb, and exhale through your left nostril. Continue alternating nostrils for several rounds of breath.

2. Tapping   https://www.youtube.com/ watch?v=pAclBdj20ZU

3. Connecting with your Shadow aspect and Shakti Mudra https://youtu.be/molK9sONMKw?si=FV6PVI23-kyFVcIA

Shakti Mudra: This mudra is said to help awaken the energy of the womb and promote healing. To do this mudra, sit comfortably with your hands on your knees. Touch the tips of your ring fingers and thumbs together, and extend your other fingers outwards.

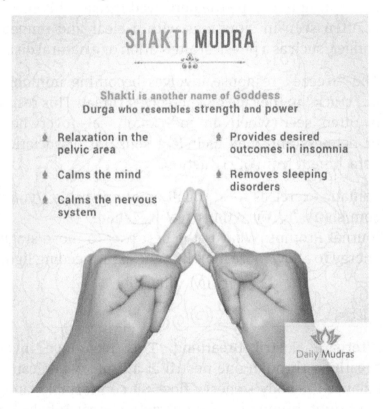

SHAKTI MUDRA

Shakti is another name of Goddess Durga who resembles strength and power

- Relaxation in the pelvic area
- Calms the mind
- Calms the nervous system
- Provides desired outcomes in insomnia
- Removes sleeping disorders

Daily Mudras

4. Journal Prompt: What benefit do I get from staying where I am?

DAY 11

1. Massage or Yin Yoga Without Props - Full Body Yin Yoga for Beginners https://youtu.be/3YOYyQ8cb5c?si=3Y_xkJMqIRlbPwuG

2. Prana Mudra: This mudra is said to help balance the body's energy and promote vitality. To do this mudra, sit comfortably with your hands on your knees. Touch the tips of your ring fingers and little fingers to the tip of your thumb, and extend your other fingers outwards.

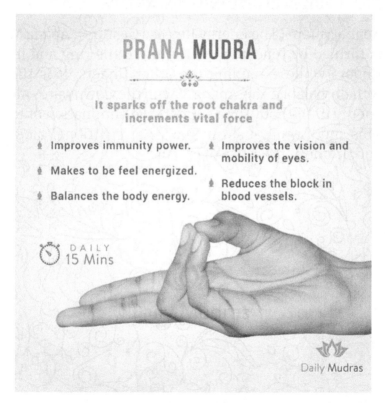

3. Pelvic Floor exercise https://www.youtube.com/watch?v=XFFDWwQgIRM

4. Journal Prompt: What triggers me about others and causes comparison or competition?

DAY 12

1. Somatic practice to move grief https://youtu.be/se3Z3GoWCG8

2. Authentic movement: This involves expressing emotions and releasing tension. The practice consists of moving the body freely and spontaneously, without judgment or preconceived notions of what the movement should look like.

Can also do a fun body-tapping movement https://www.youtube.com/watch?v=7JScerGmWrw&t=6s

3. Apana Mudra (The Energy Release Gesture): Apana Mudra is formed by touching the thumb to the ring and middle fingers while extending the other fingers. It is thought to help balance the Apana Vayu (the downward-moving energy in the body) and support the elimination of toxins. This mudra may help in releasing emotional blockages and promoting a sense of calmness.

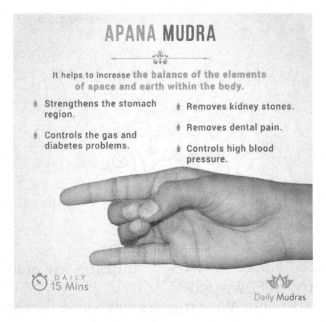

APANA MUDRA

It helps to increase the balance of the elements of space and earth within the body.

- Strengthens the stomach region.
- Controls the gas and diabetes problems.
- Removes kidney stones.
- Removes dental pain.
- Controls high blood pressure.

DAILY 15 Mins

Daily Mudras

4. Journal Prompt: What makes me want to run or leave situations?

DAY 13

1. Primordial Coding Meditation https://youtu.be/XkDMzpR53VU
2. Chakra affirmations:

   - Root Chakra– I am thriving.
   - Sacral Chakra– I am creative.
   - Solar Plexus Chakra– I am abundant.
   - Heart Chakra– I am loving.
   - Throat Chakra– I am grateful.
   - Third Eye Chakra– I am aware.
   - Crown Chakra– I am joy.

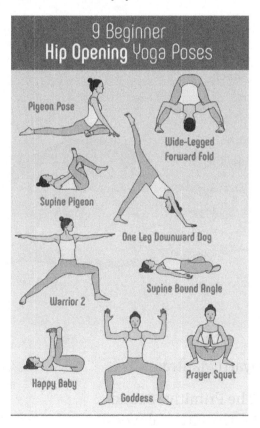

3. Hip opening poses to practice opening up the energy flow
4. Journal Prompt: What makes me angry at myself or others?

DAY 14

1. Self-led Meditation with Varuna Mudra (The Water Gesture): Varuna Mudra is formed by touching the tips of the pinky finger and thumb while extending the other fingers. It is believed to balance the water element in the body and help regulate bodily fluids. This mudra may help in promoting emotional stability and releasing emotional blockages.

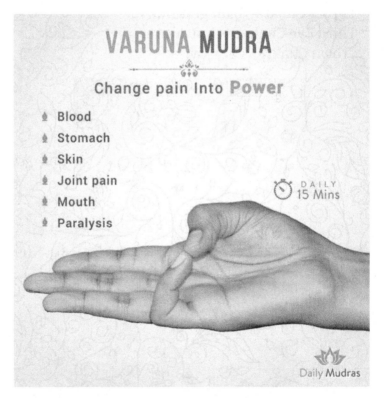

2. Chant Gayatri Mantra:

    *   Om - The Primitive Sound
    *   BHUR - The Physical World
    *   Bhuva - The mental world
    *   Svaha - The spiritual world
    *   Tat - That, God, Transcendental Paramatma

- Savitur - The Sun, The Creator, The Preserver
- Varenyam - More adorable, lovely
- Bhargo - Shine, effulgence
- Devasya - Resplendent, supreme Lord
- Deemahi - we meditate on
- Dhiyo - intelligence, understanding, Intellect
- Nah - our
- Prachadayat- enlighten, guide, inspire
- h t t p s : / / y o u t u . b e / UlnHON3tAXo?si=w5Fpa4qJFME1lMpN

3. Sound healing https://youtu.be/FDuDgCZyGUg
4. Journal Prompt: Where do I love myself deeply? Can I love all parts of me as deeply? Where are there some parts that I push down or ignore?

DAY 15

1. Mindful Self-Compassion: This practice involves bringing conscious awareness to your emotions and offering yourself kindness and support. When you notice a difficult emotion or thought, take a few moments to acknowledge it and offer yourself kind words of support, such as "May I be kind to myself at this moment. May I give myself the compassion I need?"
2. 3 min Neck & Shoulder Yoga Release (NECK & SHOULDER STRETCHES)

   https://youtu.be/KL7H9R0i2n8?si=GXT5YKJ_5mbMWWK0

3. Tapping   https://www.youtube.com/ watch?v=pAclBdj20ZU
4. Journal Prompt: Where do I feel like I shine?

DAY 16

1. Mindful Breathing: This technique involves bringing your full attention to your breath, noticing the sensation of the air moving in and out of your body. Sit in a comfortable position with your eyes closed, and focus on your breath for a few minutes. If your mind wanders, gently bring your attention back to your breath.
2. Tai Chi is a gentle, low-impact exercise involving slow, flowing movements and deep breathing. It has been shown to reduce stress and improve balance and flexibility. https://youtu.be/6w7IS8_UzHM
3. Crystal healing either with a physical crystal or an imagined one. Hold the energy of the crystal of choice and connect with the energy to assist in moving density.
4. Journal Prompt: Where do I feel like I could improve?

DAY 17

1. Practice the 'Sway Test.'

    The sway test is muscle testing often used in alternative and complementary medicine practices to assess the body's response to various stimuli. It is sometimes called the "body sway method" or "body dowsing." During the sway test, you stand upright with your feet shoulder-width apart and arms extended to the sides. Observe the body to see if it sways forward or backward in response to a yes-no question. Forward is 'yes,' and back is 'no.'

https://youtu.be/0bCf4OUaiM4

2. Eat something fresh and colorful, or have a nice warm herbal tea.
3. How To Release Blockages With Flow Training https://www.youtube.com/watch?v=HhYC2QPd7a8
4. Journal Prompt: Write your mom and dad a letter saying everything you always wanted to say (angry, sad, etc.) but never did.

DAY 18

1. Practice muscle testing https://youtu.be/Ol2vC27AMvs
2. Body Scan Meditation: This technique involves bringing your attention to different body parts, one at a time, and noticing any sensations or tension you may be holding. Lie down in a comfortable position, close your eyes, and bring your attention to your toes. Move your attention slowly up your body, noticing each part.
3. Solar code transmission meditation https://youtu.be/_UaSiNmVlQo
4. Journal Prompt: Write a letter to your womb and ask what it needs to heal.

'

DAY 19

1. Clair Gift exercise with playing cards and or matching cards if you have them (important to understand clearing of energy, having a good baseline, and good spiritual hygiene practices that can include sage, grounding, meditation, singing bowls, and energy clearing practices such as saying out loud I am clear three times until you feel the energy shift) https://youtu.be/kMTrswC8Jic
2. Walking meditation (walking in a present state where you are not thinking about the past or the future. Focus on your surroundings and really connect with the elements and nature.
3. Dance (until you lose yourself a bit and just feel the music moving you)
4. Journal Prompt: What can be cleared from my childhood or past lives?

DAY 20

1. Pendulum practice either with a necklace or pendulum (important to program and understand programming and clearing before using this tool; see video https://youtu.be/aDuk5fT6O4M
2. Pelvic Floor exercise https://youtu.be/-1lViRMMdJg
3. Yoga https://youtu.be/dtd0efI-w00
4. Journal Prompt: What needs to be cleared from past lives or versions of myself that I have outgrown?

DAY 21

1. Oracle card pull or any gift-strengthening exercise from a previous day. (Suggested cards are in the QR code if you want to order a deck.)

   - Sacred Forest
   - https://amzn.to/3RvVpqy
   - Dragon Oracle cards
   - https://amzn.to/3RvViv8
   - Earth Warriors
   - https://amzn.to/44Qwl0J
   - The Light Seer's Tarot
   - https://amzn.to/3Znmbn5
   - The Rider Tarot Deck
   - https://amzn.to/3QA7tpX
   - The Ultimate Guide to Tarot
   - https://amzn.to/478MMa3

2. Start a dream journal and listen to the Dream Enhancer meditation with Gyan Mudra https://youtu.be/5EBpXPYo8uw.

Gyan Mudra is created by touching the tip of the thumb to the tip of the index finger while keeping the other fingers extended. This mudra is known for promoting mental clarity, concentration, and inner wisdom. By calming the mind, it may indirectly support emotional well-being.

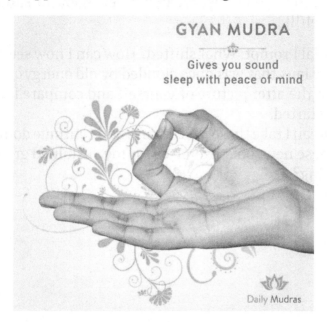

3. Myofascial release (using a rolled-up towel or roller) and eat something orange (associated with the sacral chakra color).

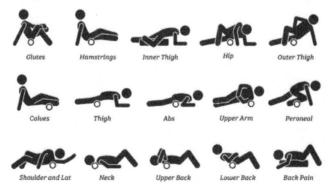

4. Journal Prompt: How can I create my best future with the strengths I have gained?

DAY 22

Congratulations, you just created a new habit of showing up for yourself!!!

1. Journal Prompt: What shifted? How can I now see through a new lens that was once clouded by old energy?
2. Paint the after picture of yourself and compare it to when you started.
3. How can I take these past 21 days and continue doing many of these new tools/exercises for my sustained growth and healing?

CHAPTER 5
DETOX, HERBS, AND NUTRITION

Before we get into the healing work, I wanted to share the nutritional piece. I learned about the importance of detoxing the body from parasites and heavy metals later in my journey, and I wish I had known sooner. Detoxing can also bring up emotion and fatigue but helps speed up the process of clearing out density and bringing in a more accurate and clear channel to your higher self and source.

SUPPLEMENTS TO SUPPORT WOMB HEALING AND HORMONE BALANCING

Several supplements and herbs are commonly used for womb healing and hormone balancing. Here are some of them:

Raspberry Leaf: Raspberry leaf has been used for centuries to support women's reproductive health. It is believed to tone the uterus, regulate menstrual cycles, and support fertility. It is commonly consumed as tea.

Dong Quai: Dong Quai is a traditional Chinese herb that supports female reproductive health. It is thought to help regulate menstrual cycles, reduce menstrual cramps, and support fertility.

Chaste Tree Berry: Also known as Vitex, this herb is commonly used to balance hormones and support menstrual health. It may help regulate menstrual cycles, reduce symptoms of PMS (premenstrual syndrome), and support fertility.

Black Cohosh: Black Cohosh is an herb traditionally used to support women's reproductive health. It often relieves menstrual cramps, regulates menstrual cycles, and helps menopausal symptoms.

Lady's Mantle: Lady's Mantle is an herb traditionally used to support uterine health and regulate menstrual cycles. It is believed to have astringent properties that can help tone the uterus and reduce excessive bleeding.

Nettle Leaf: Nettle leaf is a nutrient-rich herb often used to support overall health and well-being. It is high in vitamins and minerals that can help reproductive health and nourish the body.

Vitex: Vitex is a popular herb for balancing hormones and regulating menstrual cycles. It is commonly used to support fertility, relieve PMS symptoms, and ease menstrual cramps.

Maca Root: Maca root is an adaptogenic herb that can help balance hormones and support reproductive health. It is rich in nutrients that support hormone production and can help regulate menstrual cycles.

Black Cohosh: Black Cohosh is a herb commonly used to relieve menopause symptoms, such as hot flashes and night sweats. It is thought to help balance hormones and support reproductive health in women.

Evening Primrose Oil: Evening Primrose Oil is a rich source of gamma-linolenic acid (GLA), an essential fatty acid that can help regulate hormones and support reproductive health. It is commonly used to relieve PMS symptoms and support fertility.

It's important to note that while these supplements and herbs may be helpful for some women, they may only be appropriate for some. I have not taken all of these, but I wanted to include them as hormone health is important.

Another good resource is checking out the book "The Hormone Cure: Reclaim Balance, Sleep, Sex Drive, and Vitality Naturally with the Gottfried Protocol" by Dr. Sara Gottfried.

https://amzn.to/49nmUJJ

The concept of "detoxing" the body is widespread and can be beneficial in clearing density. Some lifestyle changes can support these processes and help the body eliminate toxins more effectively. Here are some tips:

1. *Stay hydrated*: Drinking enough water helps flush out toxins from the body and keep your bodily systems functioning optimally. Aim for at least 8-10 glasses of water per day.
2. *Eat a healthy diet*: Eating a diet rich in fruits, vegetables, whole grains, and lean proteins can help provide the necessary nutrients and antioxidants for the body to function properly and eliminate toxins.
3. *Avoid processed foods and added sugars*: Processed foods (including fake meats and cheeses), refined sugars, and artificial additives can stress the liver and other organs of elimination, making it harder for the body to detoxify.
4. *Get regular exercise*: Exercise helps to increase blood flow and oxygenation to the body's tissues, which can help to support the body's natural detoxification systems.
5. *Get enough sleep*: Sleep is critical for the body to repair and regenerate, and lack of sleep can affect the body's ability to detoxify.
6. *Reduce stress*: Chronic stress can put extra strain on the body's organs of elimination, so finding ways to manage stress, such as meditation, yoga, or deep breathing exercises, can be helpful.

These tips are the initial ways to start assisting your body in regeneration and health, allowing you to relax and become more balanced.

POPULAR DETOX FOODS

Leafy greens: Greens like spinach, kale, and arugula are rich in chlorophyll, which can help to eliminate toxins from the body. Avocado can also aid in digestion and detoxification.

Cruciferous vegetables: Vegetables like broccoli, cauliflower, and Brussels sprouts are high in sulfur-containing compounds, which can support liver function and help to eliminate toxins.

Berries: Berries like strawberries, blueberries, and raspberries are high in antioxidants, which can help to protect the body from free radical damage and support the body's natural detoxification processes.

Turmeric: Turmeric contains a compound called curcumin, which can help to reduce inflammation and support liver function.

Ginger: Ginger is a natural anti-inflammatory and can help to support digestion.

Citrus fruits: Citrus fruits like oranges, lemons, and grapefruits are high in vitamin C, which can help to support liver function and boost the immune system.

Melons: Can thoroughly cleanse the large and small intestines.

Nuts and seeds: Almonds, walnuts, pistachios, cashews, pumpkin seeds, pecans, brazil nuts, and sunflower seeds have healthy fats, fibers, vitamins, and minerals.

DECALCIFYING THE PINEAL GLAND

The pineal gland is a small endocrine gland in the brain that produces the hormone melatonin, which regulates sleep patterns. It has been called the seat of the soul.

This gland can become calcified or hardened due to various factors, such as exposure to fluoride, dietary choices, and environmental toxins. This calcification is believed to inhibit the pineal gland's function and limit its potential for spiritual experiences and consciousness expansion.

Our connection to the higher dimensional frequencies is directly related to our pineal gland. When our pineal gland is calcified, we are disconnected from our source and authentic selves. This is why the pineal gland is integral to spiritual growth and healing.

SYMPTOMS OF A CALCIFIED PINEAL GLAND

1. You may feel like you're struggling to connect to your intuition.
2. Are you having trouble making decisions? Do you rely more on facts or trust your gut feeling?
3. You wonder why you're not sleeping well and have less energy during the day.
4. You don't have dreams, or if you dream, you don't remember them.
5. You feel fearful, mistrusting, less confident, and even bored or frustrated.
6. You have uneasiness or fear around some people, experiences, and places.
7. You don't feel grounded and safe.
8. If you're empathic or intuitive, you feel like you want more but struggle to get clear and tap into intuitive gifts.
9. Attraction to nature, crystals, plants, and even oracle cards is common, but you rely so much on wisdom outside

yourself, asking others for advice rather than becoming clear.

10. Headaches, ringing in the ears, neck pain, and heightened sensitivity to chemicals and toxins plague you.
11. You struggle with your imagination, and creative ideas don't seem to flow as easily as you'd like.
12. You may have disease symptoms, feel slightly off, or feel unwell.

A HEALTHY PINEAL GLAND

A healthy pineal gland is responsible for secreting two vital brain fluids related to mental health. Those are melatonin, the hormone that induces sleep and relaxation, and serotonin, which stimulates a happy, healthy, balanced mental state.

Melatonin is produced by the pineal gland, controlling our circadian rhythms and reproductive hormones. This makes the pineal a master time regulator, affecting our sleep patterns and sexual maturation. More than just sleep-regulating, the melatonin release also affects our stress and ability to adapt to a changing world. Our happiness and well-being are directly affected by harmony in the pineal.

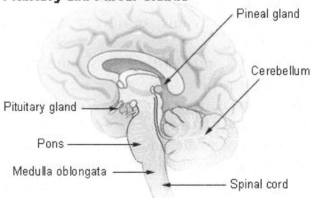

Pituitary and Pineal Glands

Pineal gland

Cerebellum

Pituitary gland

Pons

Medulla oblongata

Spinal cord

In the days of ancient Egypt, when psychic development was at its peak, specific pineal exercises were developed. Rather than being the size of a pea, it's told that the pineal gland was the size of a peach!

Consider the Eye of Horus—a literal depiction of the pineal gland resting inside the human brain. The Egyptians, Mayans, Kahunas, and others are still showing us the traditional ways to work with our third eye if we can decipher the ancient cues.

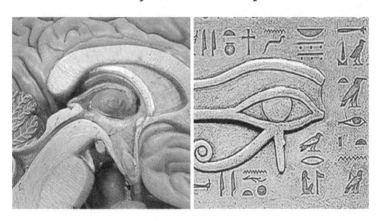

Side-by-side comparison of the Eye of Ra and a cross-section of the brain where the pineal is located

Here are ways to decalcify your pineal gland and detox your body:

1. *Reduce exposure to environmental toxins*: EMF protectors are helpful. Some environmental toxins, such as fluoride (in toothpaste and tap water), chlorine (tap water), and aluminum (deodorant and tin foil), may accumulate in the pineal gland over time. Reducing exposure to these toxins promotes overall health.
2. *Detoxification practices*: Some detoxification practices, such as infrared sauna therapy, may help to eliminate toxins from the body, including the pineal gland.
3. *Dietary changes*: A healthy diet free from processed foods and high in antioxidants helps promote the pineal gland's

health. Additionally, avoiding foods and beverages that contain fluoride can also be helpful.
4. *Meditation and mindfulness practices*: Some practitioners believe that meditation and mindfulness practices can help to activate the pineal gland and promote its overall health.
5. *Sunlight exposure*: Exposure to sunlight, particularly in the morning, can help to regulate the production of melatonin (better sleep), which is produced by the pineal gland.

FASTING

Fasting and intermittent fasting have been associated with several potential health benefits and help create a clear channel to the higher dimensional realms. I do intermittent fasting daily.

Improved insulin sensitivity: Intermittent fasting has been shown to improve insulin sensitivity, which is beneficial for blood sugar control. It may help lower blood glucose levels, reduce insulin resistance, and potentially decrease the risk of type 2 diabetes.

Reduced inflammation: Some studies suggest that intermittent fasting can lead to reduced inflammation in the body. Chronic inflammation has been linked to various health issues, including heart disease, cancer, and neurodegenerative diseases. By reducing inflammation, intermittent fasting may have potential benefits for overall health.

Enhanced cellular repair: Fasting triggers a cellular process called autophagy, which is the body's way of recycling and removing damaged cells and cellular components. Autophagy plays a role in cellular repair and may affect longevity and disease prevention.

Heart health: Intermittent fasting may have positive effects on heart health by reducing certain risk factors. It may help lower blood pressure, improve cholesterol levels, and decrease triglyceride levels, all of which are important for cardiovascular health.

Brain health: Some studies suggest intermittent fasting may have neuroprotective effects and promote brain health. It may enhance cognitive function, improve memory, and protect against neurodegenerative diseases such as Alzheimer's and Parkinson's disease. However, more research is needed in this area.

PARASITE AND HEAVY METAL INFORMATION AND CLEANSES

After working with a naturopath, I have noticed significant changes in myself following Dr. Morse's protocol for herbs.

https://morses.tv/library/

https://drmorses.com/?sca_ref=5185303.clkdik2nLZ

Below is a book I saw on a podcast. The author stated that every issue in the USA can be traced back to a parasite. The second two links are parasite cleanses, which I have done in the past.

Parasites inside me (A true story)

https://amzn.to/3rzFqxk

https://drjasondean.net/protocol

https://www.rogershood.com/product/the-parafy-kit/

IV Chelation therapy

Medical treatment involves administering chelating agents to remove heavy metals or minerals from the body. Chelation therapy is primarily used for the treatment of heavy metal poisoning, particularly lead poisoning. It may also be used as an alternative therapy for specific conditions associated with excessive heavy metal accumulation, such as mercury toxicity or iron overload in conditions like thalassemia. While I have not done this, it is an advanced protocol that is available.

CHAPTER 6

HEALING PRACTICES FOR THE WOMB

CRYSTALS

Crystals have been used for centuries for their purported healing properties, and some people believe that certain crystals can support womb healing and overall reproductive health. Here are some commonly recommended crystals for this purpose:

Moonstone: Moonstone is a popular crystal for reproductive health and is said to help balance hormones and regulate menstrual cycles.

Rose quartz: Rose quartz is associated with love and emotional healing and is sometimes used to support fertility and ease menstrual cramps.

Carnelian: Carnelian is said to help improve circulation and boost energy, which may help support reproductive health.

Black tourmaline: Black tourmaline is associated with grounding and protection, and some people use it for emotional healing and to release negative energy related to past experiences.

Bloodstone: Bloodstone is sometimes used for menstrual issues, including cramps and heavy bleeding.

When you find a crystal that calls to you, you can purchase it and cleanse it (with sage or palo santo). Then, you can set an intention with it, feel its energy and what it says to you, then place the crystal on your womb (below your belly button) as you lie down. This can help you connect with the crystal and ask for its assistance in healing your womb.

I like to pick crystals intuitively. I encourage you to work with what feels right. They will change over time as you heal. Crystals love jobs. They can be programmed to help you on your journey.

MINDFULNESS AND MEDITATION TECHNIQUES ARE THE FOUNDATION TO START THE HEALING PROCESS.

1. Mindful Breathing: This technique involves bringing your full attention to your breath, noticing the sensation of the air moving in and out of your body. Sit in a comfortable position with your eyes closed, and focus on your breath for a few minutes. If your mind wanders, gently bring your attention back to your breath.

2. Body Scan Meditation: This technique involves bringing your attention to different body parts, one at a time, and noticing any sensations or tension you may be holding. Lie down in a comfortable position, close your eyes, and bring your attention to your toes. Move your attention slowly up your body, noticing each part.

3. Loving-Kindness Meditation: This technique involves cultivating love, kindness, and compassion towards yourself and others. Sit in a comfortable position with your eyes closed, and silently repeat phrases such as "May I be happy, may I be healthy, may I be at peace" or "May you be happy, may you be healthy, may you be at peace."

4. Walking Meditation: This technique involves bringing your attention to the physical sensations of walking, such as the movement of your feet and the feeling of the ground

beneath you. Walk slowly and deliberately, focusing on your body and surroundings.

5. Guided Imagery: This technique can help to reduce stress and promote relaxation. Sit or lie comfortably, and imagine a healing light or energy surrounding your womb. Visualize this healing energy filling your body and bringing balance and harmony to your reproductive system.

6. Mindful Eating: This technique involves bringing your full attention to the eating experience and noticing your food's taste, texture, and smell. Take small bites, chew slowly, and pay attention to the sensations in your body as you eat.

Remember, mindfulness and meditation are practices that require regular effort and patience. Start with just a few minutes daily, and gradually increase the length of your practice as you become more comfortable.

I offer many guided meditation links on my YouTube channel to assist you in your mindfulness and meditation practice, including these areas: (https://www.youtube.com/channel/UClzZuzFm0wFEcUXgx6Nsigg)

1. Higher self-connection
2. Inner child
3. Womb chakra activation
4. Sacred Flame Healing
5. Shadow connection

NERVOUS SYSTEM REGULATION

Nervous system regulation and feeling safe are crucial to helping the body move through the healing journey. Many of the following exercises will help to balance the body. I found this out later in my healing journey, but it would have been really beneficial had I initially understood the importance of a balanced nervous system. Understanding the nervous system's role before doing any healing work will help tremendously with the process.

The vagus nerve, the tenth cranial nerve, is the longest in the body and plays a critical role in the autonomic nervous system. It is responsible for many essential functions, including regulating heart rate, breathing, digestion, and immune system responses. It also plays a role in emotional regulation and stress response. Stimulating the vagus nerve can have a calming effect on the body and may help reduce stress and anxiety. (*Many examples below help regulate the nervous system; others can be found online.*)

I did one session and felt so grounded and center in! My energy shifted immediately.

NERVOUS SYSTEM PRACTICES

1. Vagus Nerve reset with eye movement

   Basic exercise by Stanley Rosen

   https://www.youtube.com/watch?v=dKBEqL4PZvQ

2. Three other nervous system exercises and a short description of what happens when not regulated.

   https://www.youtube.com/watch?v=L1HCG3BGK8I&t=2s

3. Some yoga practices involve slow, controlled eye movements while holding certain postures, such as Trataka or the "gazing meditation." This practice involves staring at a single point, such as a candle flame, without blinking for several minutes. This can help improve concentration, calm the mind, and promote relaxation.

4. Similarly, some qigong practices involve gentle head and eye movements while standing or sitting in a relaxed posture. These movements are designed to promote the flow of "qi" or life force energy through the body, which can help regulate the nervous system and promote relaxation.

   https://youtu.be/y2RAEnWreoE

5. Deep breathing: Slow, deep breathing can activate the parasympathetic nervous system, which helps promote relaxation. Try to take slow, deep breaths in through your nose and out through your mouth, focusing on filling your lungs completely with each inhale and exhale.

6. Meditation: Meditation can help calm the mind and reduce stress and anxiety. There are many different types of meditation, but a simple technique is to focus on your breath, noticing each inhale and exhale and bringing your attention back to your breath each time your mind wanders.

7. Yoga: Yoga combines physical movement with breathwork and meditation, making it a great way to regulate the nervous system. Many yoga poses are designed to promote relaxation and reduce stress.

8. Tai Chi: Tai Chi is a gentle, low-impact exercise that involves slow, flowing movements and deep breathing. It has been shown to reduce stress and improve balance and flexibility.

9. Exercise: Regular physical activity can help regulate the nervous system and reduce stress. Any type of exercise that you enjoy, whether it's walking, running, swimming, or dancing, can be beneficial.

YOGA

Here are some yoga poses believed to be helpful for womb healing modifications that may be needed.:

1. Cobbler's Pose (Baddha Konasana): This pose can help to open up the hips and pelvic area, which can help to increase blood flow to the reproductive organs. Sit on the floor with the soles of your feet together and your knees bent out to the sides. Hold onto your ankles or feet with your hands, and gently press your knees towards the floor.

How to do Cobbler's Pose

yogabycandace.com

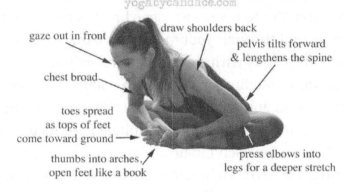

gaze out in front

draw shoulders back

pelvis tilts forward & lengthens the spine

chest broad

toes spread as tops of feet come toward ground

thumbs into arches, open feet like a book

press elbows into legs for a deeper stretch

2. Goddess Pose (Utkata Konasana): This pose is similar to a squat and can help to strengthen the pelvic floor muscles. Stand with your feet about hip-distance apart, and turn your toes out to the sides. Bend your knees and lower your hips towards the floor, keeping your spine straight and your chest lifted.

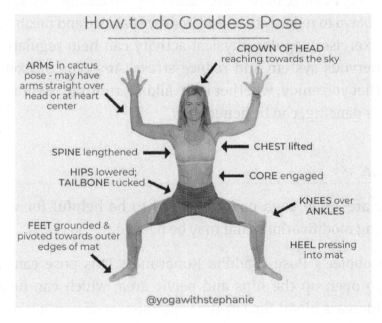

How to do Goddess Pose

CROWN OF HEAD
reaching towards the sky

ARMS in cactus pose - may have arms straight over head or at heart center

SPINE lengthened

CHEST lifted

HIPS lowered; TAILBONE tucked

CORE engaged

KNEES over ANKLES

FEET grounded & pivoted towards outer edges of mat

HEEL pressing into mat

@yogawithstephanie

3. Reclining Bound Angle Pose (Supta Baddha Konasana): This pose can help to release tension in the hips and pelvic

area and can also help to reduce stress and anxiety. Lie on your back with the soles of your feet together and your knees bent out to the sides. Place your hands on your lower abdomen and focus on deep breathing.

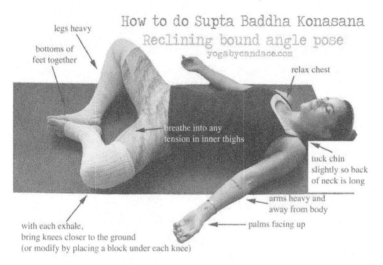

How to do Supta Baddha Konasana
Reclining bound angle pose
yogabycandace.com

legs heavy

bottoms of feet together

relax chest

breathe into any tension in inner thighs

tuck chin slightly so back of neck is long

arms heavy and away from body

with each exhale, bring knees closer to the ground (or modify by placing a block under each knee)

palms facing up

4. Camel Pose (Ustrasana): This pose can help to stretch the front of the body, including the abdomen and pelvic area.

Kneel on the floor with your knees hip-distance apart, and place your hands on your lower back. Gently arch your back and lift your chest towards the ceiling, keeping your neck neutral.

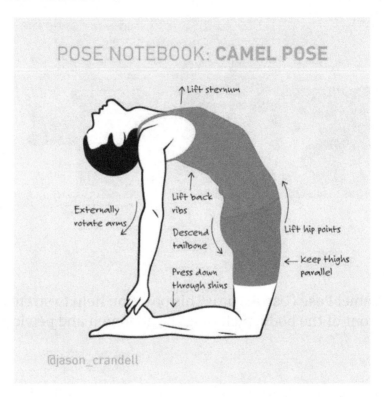

POSE NOTEBOOK: **CAMEL POSE**

↑ Lift sternum

Lift back ribs

Externally rotate arms

Descend tailbone

Lift hip points

Press down through shins

← Keep thighs parallel

@jason_crandell

5. Child's Pose (Balasana): This pose can help to relax the

body and reduce stress and tension. Kneel on the floor and sit back on your heels, then fold forward and stretch your arms out in front of you. Rest your forehead on the floor and focus on deep breathing.

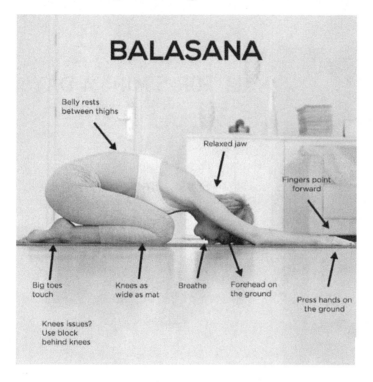

6. Legs Up the Wall Pose (Viparita Karani): This restorative

yoga pose can help promote relaxation and increase blood flow to the pelvic area. Lie on your back with your hips close to a wall, and extend your legs up the wall. Rest your arms by your sides and focus on deep breathing.

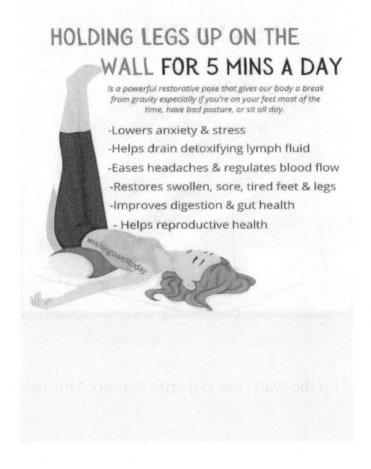

HOLDING LEGS UP ON THE WALL **FOR 5 MINS A DAY**

Is a powerful restorative pose that gives our body a break from gravity especially if you're on your feet most of the time, have bad posture, or sit all day.

-Lowers anxiety & stress

-Helps drain detoxifying lymph fluid

-Eases headaches & regulates blood flow

-Restores swollen, sore, tired feet & legs

-Improves digestion & gut health

- Helps reproductive health

7. Cat-Cow Stretch: This gentle yoga sequence can help release pelvic tension and promote relaxation. Come onto your hands and knees, with your wrists directly under your shoulders and your knees under your hips. Inhale and lift your tailbone and head towards the ceiling, allowing your belly to drop towards the floor (cow pose). Exhale and round your spine, tucking your chin towards your chest and drawing your belly button towards your spine (cat pose). Repeat for several rounds of breath.

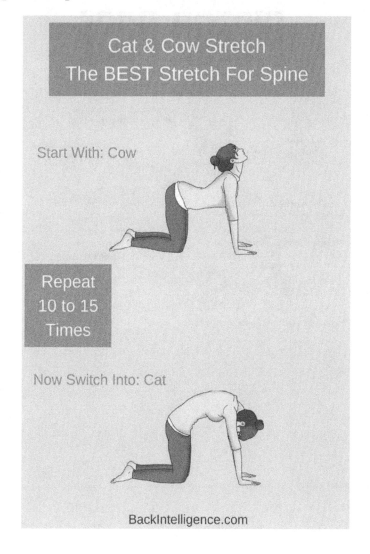

Cat & Cow Stretch
The BEST Stretch For Spine

Start With: Cow

Repeat
10 to 15
Times

Now Switch Into: Cat

BackIntelligence.com

Hip opening exercises - are beneficial for womb healing and moving energetic density out of them.

8. Pigeon pose: Start on all fours and slide one knee forward, placing it behind the opposite wrist. Extend the other leg straight back behind you, and lower your body down onto your forearms or a block. Hold for 5-10 deep breaths before switching sides.

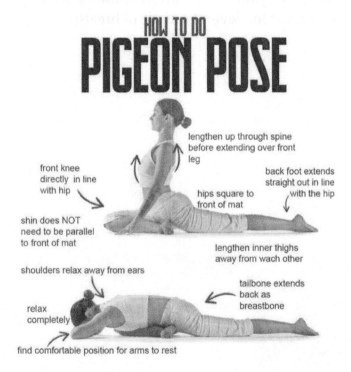

9. Butterfly pose: Sit on the floor with the soles of your feet together, knees bent out to the sides. Hold onto your ankles or feet, and gently press your knees towards the floor. Hold for 5-10 deep breaths.

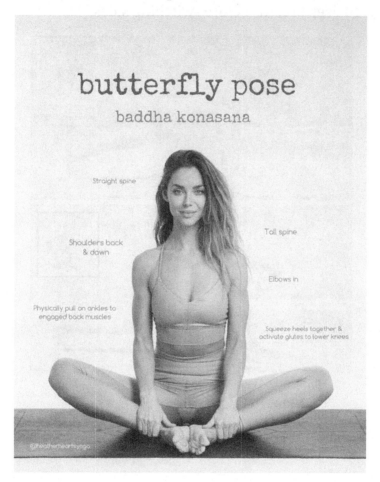

10. Lizard pose: Start in a low lunge with your right foot forward. Lower your right hand to the inside of your right foot, and walk your right foot out to the edge of your mat. Lower down onto your forearms or a block, and hold for 5-10 deep breaths before switching sides.

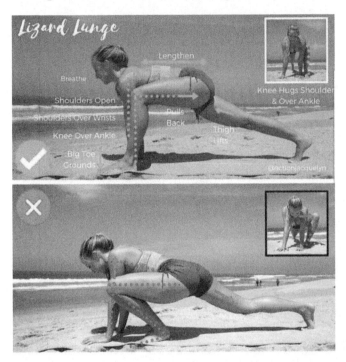

11. Bound angle pose: Sit on the floor with the soles of your feet together and knees bent out to the sides. Hold onto your ankles or feet, and gently fold forward over your legs. Hold for 5–10 deep breaths.

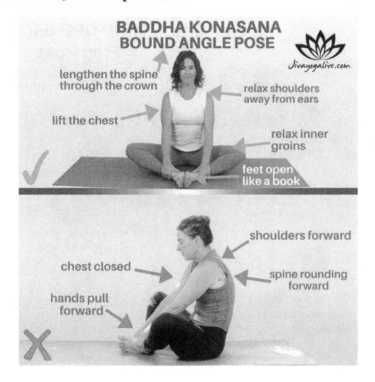

12. Frog pose: Start on all fours and slowly move your knees out to the sides, keeping your feet close together. Lower down onto your forearms or a block, and hold for 5-10 deep breaths.

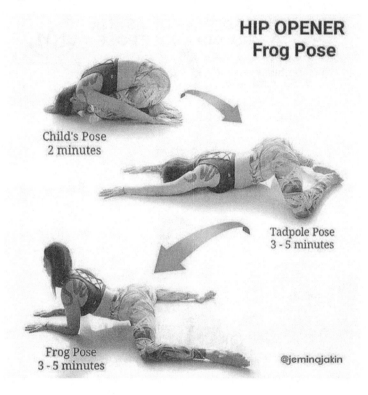

HIP OPENER
Frog Pose

Child's Pose
2 minutes

Tadpole Pose
3 - 5 minutes

Frog Pose
3 - 5 minutes

@jeminajakin

Remember, listening to your body and practicing yoga with mindfulness and intention is important. Start slow and do not push yourself; show your body love by being gentle. *If you have any health concerns or injuries, do this work with a qualified yoga teacher or healthcare practitioner before starting a new yoga practice.*

SOMATIC PRACTICES

BetterMe: Health Coaching has a 28-day somatic exercise plan or many other wall pilates and yoga plans that can help if you are new to somatic work. The focus is always slow, intentional movement.

https://apps.apple.com/us/app/betterme-health-coaching/id1264546236

Somatic practices are body-centered therapy, which focuses on the connection between the mind and body. The term "somatic" comes from the Greek word "soma," which means "the body as experienced from within." Somatic practices involve body awareness and movement to promote healing, release emotional and physical tension, and restore balance to the body. This was game-changing for me, and I do somatic exercises weekly.

The book Call of the Wild: How We Heal Trauma, Awaken Our Own Power, and Use It For Good describes the categories we can get stuck in: fit in, fawn, fight or flight, and freeze. Understanding these stages can be extremely helpful in understanding how to shift energy. These responses are part of the body's natural stress response system and are designed to help us protect ourselves in dangerous situations.

The "fit in" response involves trying to blend in with the crowd or conform to the expectations of others to avoid being noticed or singled out. This response is often seen in social situations, where an individual may feel pressure to conform to the norms and expectations of a group to avoid rejection or criticism.

The "fawn" response involves trying to please others or appease a perceived threat to avoid harm. This response is often seen in individuals who have experienced trauma or abuse and may include strategies such as people-pleasing, apologizing excessively, or avoiding conflict at all costs.

The "fight or flight" response involves confronting or attempting to escape the perceived threat. This response is often seen in situations with a clear and immediate danger, such as a physical altercation or a natural disaster.

The "freeze" response involves becoming immobilized or "stuck" in the face of a perceived threat. This response is often seen when an individual feels overwhelmed or helpless and may include a sense of dissociation or detachment from the situation.

TRAUMA RESPONSES

| FLIGHT | FIGHT | FREEZE | FAWN |

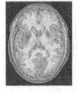 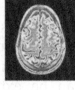 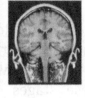 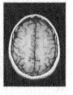

Flight	Fight	Freeze	Fawn
Workaholic	Anger	Difficulty	People
Over-thinker	outbursts	making	pleaser
Anxiety,	Controlling	decisions	Overwhelmed
panic, OCD	"The bully"	Feeling stuck	No boundaries
Difficulty	Explosive	Dissociation	Lack of
sitting still	behaviour	Isolating	identity
Perfectionist	Irritability	Numb	Codependent
Avoidance	Judgement	Shut down	Appeasing
Hyperactivity	Slamming	Exhaustion	Engaging
Sadness	doors	Indecision	self-critique
in loneliness	Self-harm	Sleeps a lot	

Understanding these different responses can help identify behavior patterns or coping mechanisms contributing to stress or anxiety. By recognizing these responses, you can begin to develop more adaptive strategies for dealing with stress and navigating difficult situations.

Call of the Wild: How We Heal Trauma, Awaken Our Own
Power, and Use It For Good

https://amzn.to/47j4MPi

Here are some examples of somatic practices:

Somatic experiencing: Somatic experiencing is a type of therapy
focusing on the connection between the body and the mind.
The goal is to help individuals release emotional and physical
tension that may be stored in the body due to traumatic
experiences. Somatic experiencing involves working with a
trained therapist to identify and release these tensions through
gentle movement and body awareness.

Authentic movement: Authentic movement involves expressing
emotions and releasing tension. The practice consists of
moving the body freely and spontaneously, without judgment
or preconceived notions of what the movement should look
like.

Dance therapy: Involves using dance and movement to promote
healing and self-expression. The practice involves working
with a trained therapist to explore emotions and release
tension through movement and dance.

FASCIA TRAUMA RELEASE

This connective tissue surrounds and supports muscles,
organs, and other structures in the body. Fascia can become
tight, restricted, or damaged due to physical trauma, injury,
poor posture, or chronic stress, leading to pain, limited range
of motion, and other discomforts.

It takes some time for the pain signal to reach the brain and
then for your brain to send out a response for you to remove
the hot item. In the meantime, your body has cells [many of
them in the fascia] that store memories faster than your brain.

Myofascial release: This technique involves applying gentle, sustained pressure on the affected area to release restrictions in the fascia. It can be done through hands-on manipulation by a skilled practitioner or by using foam rollers, balls, or other tools.

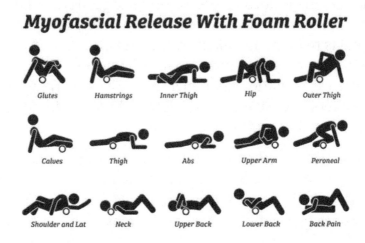

Myofascial Release With Foam Roller

Glutes Hamstrings Inner Thigh Hip Outer Thigh

Calves Thigh Abs Upper Arm Peroneal

Shoulder and Lat Neck Upper Back Lower Back Back Pain

Massage therapy: Massage techniques such as deep tissue massage, Swedish massage, or sports massage can help release tension and promote relaxation in the fascia.

Stretching and movement: Engaging in gentle stretching exercises and movement practices like yoga, Pilates, or tai chi can help improve flexibility, release tension, and promote healthy fascia.

Trigger point therapy: Trigger points are localized areas of tightness and tenderness in the muscles and fascia. Trigger point therapy involves applying pressure to these points to release tension and alleviate pain.

Instrument-assisted techniques: Specialized tools like fascia scrapers, Graston tools, or gua sha tools help break up fascial adhesions and promote healing.

Muscle Hook https://a.co/d/f0WbtX3

Fascia massage tool https://amzn.to/3RjOOzJ

Large Fascia massage tool https://amzn.to/3PHXcre

Gua Sha scraping tool https://amzn.to/3PJAXS8

Dry brushing is also good lymphatic system support and can be done in unison.

https://a.co/d/fpNIrTT

https://amzn.to/48efibD

BREATHWORK FOR WOMB HEALING

Breathwork can be a powerful tool for womb healing, as it can help increase body awareness, release tension, and promote relaxation. Here are a few breathwork techniques that may be helpful for womb healing:

https://youtu.be/ZnWufmJD7Gw?si=agrUJzIfPltE3z-M

1. *Deep Belly Breathing*: This technique involves breathing deeply into the belly, which can help to increase oxygen flow to the reproductive organs and promote relaxation. Sit or lie down in a comfortable position, and place one hand on your belly. Inhale deeply through your nose, allowing your belly to expand, and exhale fully through your mouth, allowing your belly to contract.
2. *Ujjayi Breath*: This technique is also known as "ocean breath" and involves breathing deeply through the nose while constricting the back of the throat. This can help to regulate the breath and promote relaxation. Sit or stand comfortably, inhale deeply through your nose while constricting the back of your throat. Exhale entirely through your nose, tightening the back of your throat.
3. *Alternate Nostril Breathing*: This technique involves

breathing through one nostril at a time, which can help balance the body's energy flow. Sit comfortably, and use your right thumb to close your right nostril. Inhale deeply through your left nostril, and then use your right ring finger to close your left nostril. Exhale entirely through your right nostril, and then inhale deeply through your right nostril. Close your right nostril with your thumb, and exhale through your left nostril. Continue alternating nostrils for several rounds of breath.

MUDRAS

A mudra is a symbolic hand gesture or posture used in Hinduism, Buddhism, and yoga. The word "mudra" is Sanskrit for "seal," "mark," or "gesture." Mudras are believed to help create a specific energy flow within the body and are often used in meditation, yoga, and other spiritual practices. I liked using mudras early in my meditation practices as I had difficulty sitting still. It gave me something to focus on with my hands. Holding crystals also helped quiet my mind because I could turn them and focus on the feeling of the cold stone in my hand.

Several mudras can be used for womb healing; here are a few examples:

Yoni Mudra: This mudra is also known as the "womb seal" and is said to help balance the energy of the reproductive system. To do this mudra, sit comfortably with your back straight and your hands on your knees. Bring the tips of your thumbs and index fingers together to form a triangle, and rest your hands on your lower abdomen.

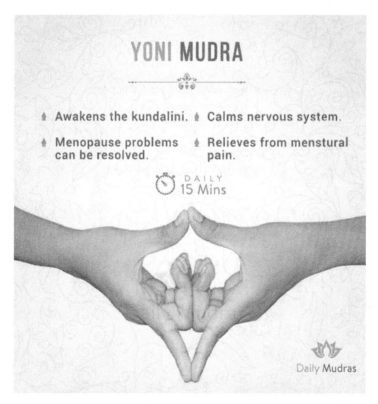

Shakti Mudra: This mudra is said to help awaken the energy of the womb and promote healing. To do this mudra, sit comfortably with your hands on your knees. Touch the tips of your ring fingers and thumbs together, and extend your other fingers outwards.

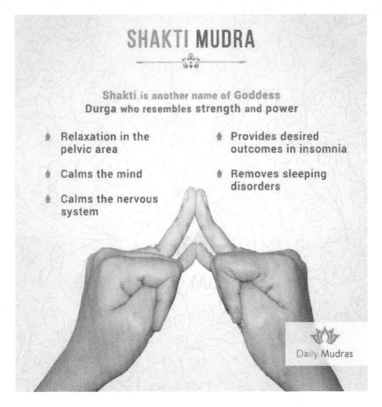

SHAKTI MUDRA

Shakti is another name of Goddess
Durga who resembles strength and power

- Relaxation in the pelvic area
- Calms the mind
- Calms the nervous system

- Provides desired outcomes in insomnia
- Removes sleeping disorders

Daily Mudras

Prana Mudra: This mudra is said to help balance the body's energy and promote vitality. To do this mudra, sit comfortably with your hands on your knees. Touch the tips of your ring fingers and little fingers to the tip of your thumb, and extend your other fingers outwards.

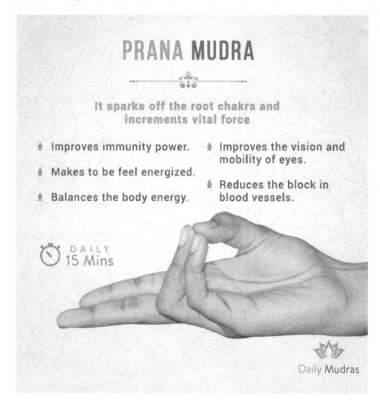

Apana Mudra (The Energy Release Gesture): Apana Mudra is formed by touching the thumb to the ring and middle fingers while extending the other fingers. It is thought to help balance the Apana Vayu (the downward-moving energy in the body) and support the elimination of toxins. This mudra may help in releasing emotional blockages and promoting a sense of calmness.

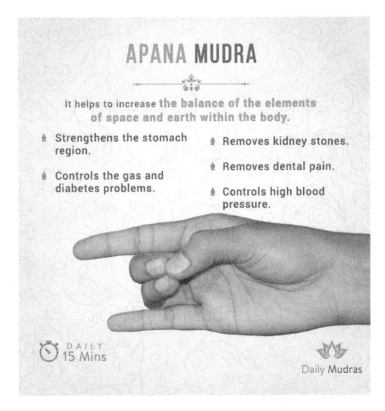

Gyan Mudra (The Knowledge Gesture): Gyan Mudra is created by touching the tip of the thumb to the tip of the index finger while keeping the other fingers extended. This mudra is known for promoting mental clarity, concentration, and inner wisdom. By calming the mind, it may indirectly support emotional well-being.

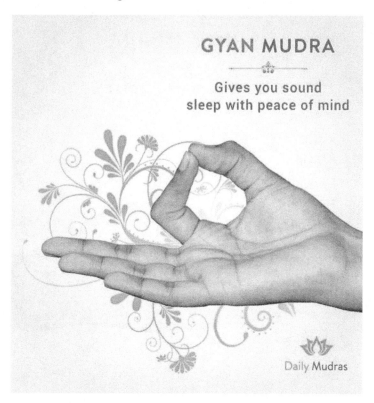

GYAN MUDRA

Gives you sound
sleep with peace of mind

Daily Mudras

Varuna Mudra (The Water Gesture): Varuna Mudra is formed by touching the tips of the pinky finger and thumb while keeping the other fingers extended. It is believed to balance the water element in the body and help regulate bodily fluids. This mudra may help in promoting emotional stability and releasing emotional blockages.

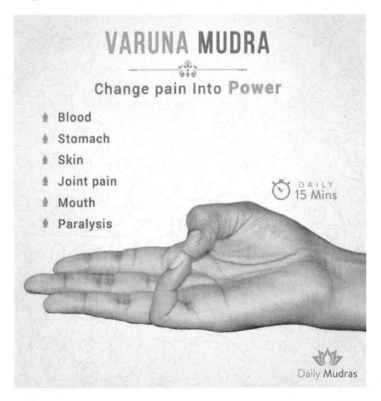

VARUNA MUDRA

Change pain Into Power

- Blood
- Stomach
- Skin
- Joint pain
- Mouth
- Paralysis

DAILY
15 Mins

Daily Mudras

CHANTING

Chanting can be a powerful tool for womb healing, as it can help calm the mind, balance the body's energy, and promote relaxation. Here are a few chants that may be helpful for womb healing:

1. *Om*: This is one of the most well-known chants in yoga and is believed to represent the sound of the universe. Chanting "om" can help to promote relaxation and balance the energy of the body. Sit in a comfortable position, close your eyes, and take a deep breath. On the exhale, chant "om" for as long as you like, allowing the sound to vibrate through your body.
2. *Gayatri Mantra*: This powerful mantra promotes healing and balance in the body and mind. Sit in a comfortable position with your eyes closed, and take a deep breath in. Chant the Gayatri Mantra: "Om Bhur Bhuvah Swaha, Tat Savitur Varenyam, Bhargo Devasya Dheemahi, Dhiyo Yo Nah Prachodayat."

Repeat the mantra for several rounds of breath. This is one of my favorite things to help bring the mind back to presence.

Om- The Primitive Sound

BHUR - The Physical World

Bhuva - The mental world

Svaha - The spiritual world

Tat - That, God, Transcendental Paramatma

Savitur - The Sun, The Creator, The preserver

Varenyam - More adorable, lovely

Bhargo - Shine, effulgence

Devasya - Resplendent, supreme Lord

Deemahi - we meditate on

Dhiyo - intelligence, understanding, Intellect

Nah - our

Prachadayat- enlighten, guide, inspire

https://youtu.be/UlnHON3tAXo?si=w5Fpa4qJFME1lMpN

CHAPTER 7

EMOTIONAL HEALING

Emotional healing refers to the process of addressing and resolving emotional wounds, traumas, and imbalances to restore emotional well-being, inner peace, and overall mental and psychological health. It involves acknowledging, understanding, and working through painful emotions, experiences, and patterns that have caused distress or hindered personal growth. Emotional healing can occur on various levels, including individual, interpersonal, and collective.

Emotional healing is important so we can learn to balance the spectrum of the emotional scale instead of getting stuck at one end or the other. Everything feeds into the body, nervous system, and spiritual maturity.

Emotional healing is vital for several reasons, as it profoundly affects us. Internally, when we don't heal our emotional body, it can cause physical issues, pain, and difficulty. Externally, it can make relationships hard and lead to projecting things onto others that have nothing to do with them. We have a limited scope of understanding when operating from an emotional trigger or wound. We don't hear the information. We just react, which can blow things out of proportion quickly. When you start working with your emotional body, you begin to see how others are reacting from wounds or fear, and it can turn into anger or lashing out, but it has nothing to do with you. Here are some key reasons why emotional healing is significant and how it can impact individuals internally and externally:

Internal Benefits:

Emotional Well-being: Emotional healing helps individuals achieve greater emotional well-being by addressing and resolving deep-seated emotional wounds, traumas, and negative patterns. It releases emotional pain, fostering inner peace and promoting a more positive emotional state.

Self-Awareness and Self-Understanding: Engaging in emotional healing work facilitates self-awareness and self-understanding. It helps individuals gain insights into their emotional triggers, patterns, and reactions, leading to a deeper understanding of oneself. This awareness promotes personal growth, self-acceptance, and the ability to make conscious choices aligned with one's values and needs.

Increased Resilience: Emotional healing enhances resilience by providing individuals with tools and skills to cope with life's challenges. It equips them with emotional resources, such as self-regulation, healthy coping mechanisms, and effective problem-solving strategies, contributing to better emotional stability and adaptability.

Improved Relationships: Emotional healing positively impacts personal relationships. By addressing and healing emotional wounds, individuals become better equipped to engage in healthier, more authentic connections. They can communicate their needs, boundaries, and emotions more effectively, improving intimacy, trust, and emotional connection with others.

Enhanced Self-Compassion and Self-Worth: Emotional healing nurtures self-compassion and self-worth. It involves acknowledging and validating one's emotions, experiences and needs without judgment. Individuals can cultivate a stronger sense of self-worth by healing past wounds and developing self-compassion, increasing self-esteem and self-confidence.

External Benefits:

Improved Communication: Emotional healing can enhance communication skills, allowing individuals to express their emotions, thoughts, and needs more effectively. Leading to healthier and more authentic interactions, reducing relationship misunderstandings and conflicts.

Conflict Resolution: Emotional healing equips individuals to navigate conflicts more constructively. It fosters empathy, understanding, and the capacity to listen and respond compassionately.

Better Boundaries: Emotional healing supports the development and maintenance of healthy boundaries. It helps individuals recognize their limits, communicate their boundaries, and assertively protect their emotional well-being. This can lead to healthier and more balanced relationships and prevent emotional overwhelm or exploitation.

Increased Empathy and Compassion: Individuals who engage in emotional healing can develop a deeper empathy and compassion towards themselves and others.

Personal and Professional Success: Emotional healing can positively impact personal and professional success. By addressing emotional wounds and limiting beliefs, individuals can overcome self-sabotaging patterns and develop a stronger sense of self-efficacy.

Overall, emotional healing is important because it allows individuals to address and heal past emotional wounds, cultivate self-awareness and self-compassion, improve relationships, and enhance overall well-being. Through this process, individuals can experience greater emotional stability, personal growth, and an improved quality of life.

Here are some key aspects and approaches to emotional healing:

TECHNIQUES FOR EMOTIONAL RELEASE.

1. *Artistic Expression*: Engaging in creative activities such as drawing, painting, or dancing can help release emotions and allow self-expression.
2. *Journaling*
3. *Self-compassion practices*
4. *Energy healing*: Can help unblock and balance the body's energy flow. (I will talk more about this later in this book.)
5. *Forgiveness*
6. *Talking*: Sometimes, simply talking through your emotions with a trusted friend can help you process and release them.

JOURNALING PROMPTS FOR WOMB HEALING

Journaling through writing down your thoughts and feelings can be a powerful way to process and release emotions. Set aside time each day to write in a journal, allowing yourself to express whatever comes up for you freely.

Here are some questions to ask yourself to build up your relationship with your womb:

What does your womb want to tell you?

Where in your body do you feel pain or discomfort when connecting with your womb space?

Where has held onto this pain, discomfort, trauma, or energy hurt you?

Where do you blame yourself or others for things in the past?

When you talk to yourself, is it positive or negative?

What does your inner child crave that she has not received?

What is the best way to heal and repair the trauma inside your body?

Where do you feel unsafe, unseen, or unheard?

What is the best way to move stagnant energy to allow more light into the areas needing light?

What benefit do you get from staying where you are?

What triggers you about others and causes comparison or competition?

What makes you want to run or leave situations?

What makes you angry?

Where do you criticize yourself?

Where do you love yourself deeply? Can you love all parts of you as deeply?

Where do you feel like you shine?

Where do you feel like you could improve?

Write a letter to your mom and or dad saying everything you always wanted to say but never did.

Write a letter to your womb and ask what it needs to heal.

What is ready to be cleared from your childhood or past lives?

What needs to be cleared from past lives or versions of yourself you have outgrown?

How can you now create your best new future out of the strengths you gained?

What shifted? How can you now see through a new lens clouded by old energy?

SELF-COMPASSION PRACTICES AND MY FAVORITE HO'OPONOPONO

Self-compassion practices involve treating yourself with kindness, empathy, and understanding, particularly in times of difficulty or stress. Here are a few self-compassion practices you may find helpful:

Self-Compassion Break: Give yourself compassion and love during a difficult emotional release. Start by placing your hand over your heart and saying, "This is not permanent but just a moment of energy shifting through me." May I be kind to myself? May I give myself the compassion I need?"

Loving-Kindness Meditation: This practice involves sending love to yourself and others. Start by sitting or lying in a comfortable position, and bring to mind a specific person, including yourself. Repeat phrases of good wishes such as "May I be happy, may I be healthy, may I be safe, may I be at peace."

Gratitude Practice: Gratitude practices can help shift your focus from negative thoughts or emotions to positive ones. Take a few moments each day to write down or reflect on things you are grateful for, such as the people in your life, experiences you've had, or something you've accomplished.

Mindful Self-Compassion: This practice involves bringing conscious awareness to your emotions and offering yourself kindness and support. When you notice a difficult emotion or thought, take a few moments to acknowledge it and offer yourself kind words of support, such as "May I be kind to myself at this moment. May I give myself the compassion I need?"

Ho'oponopono is a traditional Hawaiian practice of reconciliation and forgiveness. The word "Ho'oponopono" means "to make things right." It involves recognizing and taking responsibility for one's thoughts, actions, and emotions and seeking to make amends and restore balance. This is a practice I used for months when working on self-love.

The practice involves repeating four simple phrases: "I'm sorry, please forgive me, thank you, I love you." The idea is to use these phrases to acknowledge and take responsibility for one's thoughts and emotions and express gratitude and love towards oneself and others.

Here's how a Ho'oponopono practice might look:

Find a quiet and comfortable space where you can sit or lie down.

Consider a person or situation causing distress, discomfort, or conflict.

Repeat the phrases "I'm sorry; please forgive me, thank you, I love you" silently to yourself, directing them towards the person or situation.

Allow yourself to feel emotions like sadness, anger, or frustration. Notice any physical sensations in your body, such as tension or tightness.

Continue to repeat the phrases, allowing yourself to feel and release any emotions that arise.

When you feel ready, take a deep breath and release the phrases. Notice how you feel, and allow yourself to rest and integrate the experience.

https://youtu.be/2TePAocURL

TAPPING AND BODY TAPPING

https://www.youtube.com/watch?v=pAclBdj20ZU

https://www.youtube.com/watch?v=7JScerGmWrw&t=6s

1. Identify the issue: Start by identifying the issue or emotion that you want to address with tapping. This could be a specific fear, anxiety, or physical discomfort.
2. Rate the intensity: Rate the intensity of the issue or emotion on a scale from 0-10, with 10 being the most intense.
3. Choose a setup statement: Choose a simple statement that acknowledges the issue or emotion and affirms your self-acceptance and self-love. For example, "Even though I feel anxious, I deeply and completely love and accept myself."
4. Tap the points: Using your fingertips, tap on each of the following points while repeating your setup statement:

   - Karate chop (side of the hand)
   - Eyebrow (inner edge)
   - Side of eye
   - Under eye
   - Under nose
   - Chin
   - Collarbone
   - Under arm
   - Top of head

5. Repeat and check-in: After completing a round of tapping, take a deep breath and rate the intensity of the issue or emotion again. If it has decreased, continue tapping and repeating the process. If it hasn't decreased, adjust your setup statement and continue tapping.

Remember, listening to your body and practicing these techniques with mindfulness and intention is important. If you have difficulty processing or releasing emotions or experiencing intense or overwhelming emotions, it's important to seek support.

CHAPTER 8

INNER CHILD HEALING AND SHADOW WORK

The inner child is the child-like part in all of us. Those moments we remember when we were a child when we lit up with innocence and excitement or laughter and playful fun energy. Our inner child lives inside us even into adulthood, and understanding our inner child's needs is extremely important for the healing journey. If we don't play with our inner child and spend time enjoying life, there will be hard stops and roadblocks to the process and how we get through the healing journey. Neglecting our inner child is like ignoring a real child. There are repercussions, and your inner child is not easily forgotten for long. Things will manifest unpleasantly in the physical the longer this part of us is ignored.

<u>Working with your inner child is paramount in any type of healing work.</u> This relationship must be cultivated and nurtured. The link has a guided meditation to help you begin to work with your inner child. Like shadow integration, inner child integration is necessary to expand and heal.

Inner child Mediation

<u>https://youtu.be/ZNci8FjBKko?si=KMyRZWJpF9saCXDe</u>

Inner child healing refers to the process of addressing and healing the emotional wounds and traumas that occurred during childhood. It involves recognizing and nurturing the part of us that represents our childhood self and holds our past experiences, emotions, and beliefs. Inner child healing aims to heal and integrate the wounded inner child, allowing for emotional growth, self-compassion, and personal transformation.

Here are some ways to work with inner child healing:

Acknowledgment and connection: Inner child healing begins with recognizing and acknowledging the existence and impact of our inner child. Establishing a compassionate and nurturing relationship with the inner child is essential in healing. We will begin to see the connection to our beliefs, behaviors, and emotional patterns in adulthood.

Reparenting the Inner Child: Reparenting involves providing the love, care, and support that may have been missing during childhood. It entails meeting the inner child's needs and offering comfort, validation, and reassurance.

Healing Childhood Trauma: Inner child healing often involves addressing and healing childhood traumas or wounds. Trauma-focused therapies such as somatic experiencing, or inner child therapy can help process and release traumatic memories and emotions.

Releasing Repressed Emotions: Inner child healing allows for the safe expression and release of repressed emotions from childhood. This may involve journaling, art therapy, somatic release exercises, or talking with a trusted therapist or support group.

Revisiting and Reframing Beliefs: Exploring and reframing the limiting beliefs formed during childhood is an important aspect of inner child healing. We can replace negative thoughts with more empowering and nurturing ones by identifying and challenging negative thoughts.

Setting Boundaries and Self-Care: Inner child healing involves healthy boundaries and prioritizing self-care. We can recognize and honor our needs more quickly, saying no when necessary and engaging in activities that promote self-nurturing and well-being.

Integration and Inner Wholeness: Inner child healing aims to integrate the healed inner child with the adult self, fostering inner wholeness and emotional integration. The inner child is essential to our being and embracing their innocence, creativity, and joy.

Inner child healing is a deeply personal and transformative process that requires patience, self-compassion, and support. It is important to approach inner child healing with gentleness and respect, allowing the process to unfold naturally and comfortably.

Today, I spend most of my time being present and creating the most beautiful life. I am guided to do the heavy lifting and shadow work when ready to expand again (some call this upleveling). We may spend chunks of time processing emotion, but we must remember we are here to have fun, enjoy life, and not take things too seriously.

I spent a lot of time at the beginning of my healing journey, forgetting to have fun, and when our inner child feels neglected, we can get stuck and unable to shift out of the density. It can feel like a heavy, daunting journey where we crave an end date or just want to get through it. If we are looking for an ending, it's a sign we need to play more. The inner child can help us by reminding us of the light state of being we are meant to flow as. She can pick us up and help with integration when she is seen and acknowledged. I always say the old saying that if mama isn't happy, no one is happy, but this has never been truer for our inner child. She just wants attention and has the magic to help in more ways than one when we are conscious and attentive to her.

INNER CHILD HEALING

Sometimes, this work can entail some discomfort. You need to see your inner child. Talk to her. Sit with her. Let her be angry at you if she's mad. Let her scream and cry. Don't leave her until she is completely satisfied and feels safe. Tell her you're sorry you left her. Ask what she needs. Be sure she knows you are not leaving her again. Make sure you put her somewhere safe when you go—a space just for her. She needs to feel love and support. When trauma occurs, we lose parts of ourselves because survival mode is necessary.

When digging into inner child healing and shadow work, we can find the times we lost a part of ourselves and reintegrate it. For example, when you lose trust, security, confidence, etc., revisit the time and find your inner child who was left alone and scared. Then, if drawn to a physical part of the body, massage the area of the body. This helps dislodge the stuck energy.

Spend time with your inner child every day. Go back to the times of the trauma. Feel, sense, and imagine you are there again. Sit through the experience again. Be fully present to what is going on. When it no longer brings up emotion, you can move on. This may take a few tries.

Once you start this, find times when you lost part of yourself, and mark once she has returned. Then, move on to a different time.

Once you do this a few times, it's easier. She will show up easier when you get used to spending time with your inner child. You want to gain her trust, and that takes time to show up so she knows you won't leave her again. No blame, just forgiveness. She will start to trust you again. It may bring tears, but begin to have more fun with her. We want that little girl to regain her confidence, zest for life, and joy. Only then does your purpose unfold completely. Your eyes will open even wider.

Inner child adventures are one of my favorite activities. We go on dragon rides and explore imaginative lands. Play is also a way to nurture your inner child and remember what that inner joy feels like. Things you liked in childhood, such as creative projects, water parks, roller coasters, carnivals, and Christmas lights, can help bring her back to life. Whatever it is that makes you remember happiness and fun will be helpful with inner child relationship cultivation.

SHADOW WORK AND THE PAIN BODY

Meditation to connect with your shadow aspect

https://youtu.be/molK9sONMKw?si=Zzd419uj47gCLNzU

I spent much time at the beginning of my spiritual journey just trying to unpack trauma. Digging for things we are not ready to heal and trying to go too fast is a recipe for disaster. It slows us down and keeps us in this up-and-down yo-yo. We need balance, rest, fun, excitement, understanding, and discovering our history and who we are. We must learn to be still and work on our nervous system and physical body. Then, yes, the heavy lifting, too. But balance is critical.

Shadow Work is a term that originated from the field of psychology, particularly in the work of Carl Jung, a Swiss psychiatrist and psychoanalyst. It refers to exploring and integrating the unconscious or "shadow" aspects of one's personality.

According to Jung, the shadow represents the aspects of ourselves that we have repressed, denied, or deemed unacceptable. These can include our fears, insecurities, desires, and other qualities that we may find uncomfortable or inappropriate. The shadow is often formed during childhood due to societal conditioning, cultural influences, and personal experiences.

Engaging in shadow work involves bringing these hidden

aspects of ourselves into conscious awareness and accepting them as part of who we are. It requires a willingness to explore our inner depths, confront our fears and insecurities, and embrace our whole selves.

Shadow work can take various forms, including self-reflection, journaling, dream analysis, meditation, and therapy. It often involves identifying and acknowledging behavior patterns, exploring their origins, and working towards integration and self-acceptance.

The goal of shadow work is not to eliminate or suppress these aspects of ourselves but rather to understand and integrate them in a healthy and balanced way. Doing so can gain greater self-awareness, emotional resilience, and personal growth.

It's important to note that shadow work can be a deep and sometimes challenging process, as it may involve confronting uncomfortable truths and facing aspects of ourselves that we may have avoided. Seeking support to work through more profound trauma healing and shadow work is important. I am here to help. You don't have to do this work alone.

I feel it's crucial to understand shadow work before emerging into energy work practices.

Shadow Work is the process of bringing anything we hold unconscious to light. We need a good understanding of how the healing journey will go up and down on the emotional scale so we do not attach to one part. Each section of the emotional scale will ebb and flow.

The pain body is a term coined by spiritual teacher Eckhart Tolle to describe the accumulation of emotional pain and trauma we carry from past experiences. The pain body can become activated by triggers in our environment or interactions with others, causing us to relive past pain and react in ways not in alignment with our true selves.

Here are some steps you can take to begin shadow work and address the pain body:

1. Identify your shadows: Take time to reflect on the parts of yourself that you may have suppressed or denied. This could involve exploring your fears, insecurities, and negative self-talk.

2. Acknowledge and accept your shadows: Practice accepting and embracing these aspects of yourself without judgment or shame. Recognize that they are a natural part of being human and everyone has shadows they struggle with.

3. Explore your pain body: Pay attention to the triggers that activate your pain body, and notice how it feels in your body. Practice bringing mindful awareness to these sensations without judgment or resistance.

4. Release emotional blockages: Use practices that can help release emotional blockages, such as mindfulness meditation, breathwork, or creative expression.

There will be times when you will have discomfort as you process emotion. Understanding how to move through the density without attaching to the lower frequencies is crucial. I like to use the term "Holding space." It refers to being present for yourself without judgment, criticism, or trying to fix anything. It means creating a safe and supportive environment to express your thoughts and feelings. I repeatedly say, "You're okay," or "You're safe to feel this," as I hold my heart when discomfort comes up during processing. When working through deep trauma, you may need support.

Physical nausea and pain can arise as you are clearing energy. If you are new to this work, I recommend doing the meditations provided in this book from my YouTube channel so you can get used to connecting with your higher self and understanding how she will help guide you.

Integration of energy healing is paramount. If we do not

understand how to release and clear the layers as we go, we compound work that will have to be unpacked later.

No matter how hard the work gets, I always tell myself and others that the upswing of a new level of peace, joy, and happiness is waiting. You will know you are through a layer of processing when you physically feel the shift. You may feel lighter and more open. You may feel the energy leave your body. You may feel like you just can't cry or write anymore. We all have different Clair gifts (our psychic channel that feel, sense, see, or hear messages from our higher self). So, we will all have different experiences with how we do this work. Just know you are not alone; there is no right or wrong way to do the work.

My personal experience with shadow work has been life-changing. I have accepted parts of myself I didn't think were worth loving and found compassion and understanding for myself and others in more profound ways than I thought possible.

Sometimes, we need assistance seeing things that lurk in the dark. For example, Acacia Lawson, my editor, found my writer's block that stemmed from a childhood experience, and now this book and the others are free to come to life. We sometimes have blind spots that, no matter how much work we do, we need help seeing. But once aware, it can shift quickly and easily.

Consistency is key, as well as learning your own body and how it works.

POST INTEGRATION SHADOW WORK

Shadow work and reintegrating fragments (parts we have pushed down) into ourselves.

If the tears come, let them out. If anger comes up, let it out.

Writing is always an excellent way to release these emotions or to start the stream of them coming out. Screaming and crying will also release emotions. Deep breathing can intensify the release. This is recommended throughout this journey when doing shadow work—deep belly breathing in and out or quick breathing in and out.

Remember, the emotion doesn't have to last long. It can be as short as 1 minute. Essential oils, Sage, Palo Santo, and crystals are also helpful for this work. Often, situations and experiences occur in our lives because of our shadow, not outside causes, so we struggle with processing this or understanding the root cause.

A timeline review may be beneficial if you want to cover important things that might have been forgotten. Start when you were born and make a timeline of important events going through today. This should also include trauma and anything that sticks out, good or bad. It may not necessarily be a traumatic experience that caused the fragmentation. It could be minor, but it still had a profound effect if it stuck with you, no matter how significant or insignificant it goes on the timeline.

When you go through the list, things will stand out with a theme around what is ready to be healed first. We want to make sure the fragment gets integrated completely back in. I've done timeline reviews several times, and new things always come up. You can also see themes. Like every seven to ten years, something significant happens. Notice where you have themes, dates, months, and expansion areas throughout the year.

OTHER WAYS TO INDUCE EMOTION

There are various ways to get repressed, forgotten, or stuck emotions out of your body to heal and become lighter (mentally, physically, emotionally, and energetically).

1. Feeling into what is ready to process through timeline dates
2. Hawaiian forgiveness prayer – Ho'oponopono This can be done in the mirror or with specific people you want to forgive.
3. Mediation
4. Journaling
5. Sad music (to bring things up, I like Audiomachine and Epic Legacy Trailer Music)
6. Triggers
7. Worthiness practice and mirror work
8. Inner child healing
9. Womb healing
10. Bodywork (massage, stretching, fascia release, somatic exercise)
11. Detox and diet (trauma is stored in our fat cells and body, so diet is important for our mood and physical body while we do healing work)

SHADOW WORK PRACTICE

Be in a quiet place where you will not be disrupted. You can make this sacred with a sacred space or mantra.

Focus on one thing at a time when you had pain, felt sadness, etc., how you felt with every feeling, sensation, and emotion; don't leave any stone unturned. You can use your timeline map if you are unsure what to focus on. We call fragmentation of consciousness when we split off from a part of ourselves because something is too painful to experience. This memory/fragmentation can be from a past life as well. Once you get used to working with the current processing of emotion, many times, past lives come up to heal as well. This is usually shown in meditation.

I've had times where the same scene came to me several times for deeper layers of work. This is why I stress this so very much. To truly integrate, especially if your shadow is coming up, sit with it until it no longer hurts in your body or the tears dry up.

The second most important thing about shadow work is to avoid getting stuck. Sometimes, when we revisit certain times, thoughts, events, or energies, we can feel comfort in that space because it has been with us for so long. Being firm in the determination to shift the energy and stay in your power wasn't highlighted at the beginning of my journey. There is processing vs. feeling sorry for ourselves because XYZ has happened. We want to feel the entire range of what has been trapped or fragmented, but we do not want to stay there. Find the strength and understand we are not there anymore. Here and now is where we are needed. The strengths we gained make it easier to take the good, leave the bad, and keep it moving. Knowing you have the support and are not alone is important. If you need assistance, I can help or recommend a trusted colleague.

CHAPTER 9
SHIELDING AND PROTECTION

2017 was what some would call my 'dark night of the soul.' I had connected with my higher self enough to find the way through my fertility issues, but my gut health and nervous system were shot. If you are unfamiliar with the term 'dark night', it describes a period of intense spiritual awakening. It is often characterized by confusion, sadness, and spiritual emptiness or disconnection as you begin to see through the veil. It is named this because we can not return to the old ways after a spiritual awakening.

It may be triggered by various factors such as loss, trauma, being diagnosed with something, or the breakdown of one's beliefs or values. This was what sent me to that first healing session, as I mentioned at the beginning of this workbook, and how it brought me back to joy. I wanted that feeling back— that safety and freedom to be so in the moment and so light. As I started learning various healing modalities and how to connect with my Clair gifts, I realized it is just a spiral; we work through layers and keep evolving.

The reason I hit this low was understood better when I began to look at my childhood sexual abuse (suppressed memory retrieval later would help unpack even more understanding of this). The world we live in, the trafficking of children becoming more widely seen, was why this intense period began for me. It was pulling everything I had hidden and buried back up. I started going down the rabbit hole of why we needed energy healing to begin with. I had always questioned our existence, and I spent hours talking about how there must be more than this 9-5 life in my 20s. I began a quest back to me and to understand everything I had shut down at age 16.

While the experience of the dark night of the soul can be extremely difficult, it is a very transformative experience that can lead to greater spiritual insight or growth. Many spiritual traditions emphasize the importance of persevering through such periods of suffering better to understand oneself and one's place in the world.

I worked with a few practitioners and began learning modalities. After I was comfortable working with energy, I moved on to memory retrieval, working with multidimensional aspects, past life healing, bringing back lost soul fragments, and doing timeline work. This more high-level stuff is best done with a trusted practitioner first and with the understanding of proper shielding and protection practices before beginning solo retrievals. I can help, and if I can't help, I have trusted colleagues I send people to depending on what the person needs.

Before any kind of energy work, understanding shielding and clearing are crucial practices. You are already automatically shielded and protected in my meditations. *(This is not true with all online meditations, practitioners, and courses. Some are not here to assist the highest good.)*

Shielding and clearing energy are practices often used to protect oneself from negative energy and release any negative energy that may have accumulated in one's energy field.

Shielding involves creating a protective barrier around oneself that blocks out negative or siphoning energy. This can be done through visualization or physical objects, such as crystals or protective symbols. The intention is to create a shield that allows positive energy to flow while keeping out negative energy.

Clearing energy involves releasing negative or stagnant energy. This can be done through various methods such as meditation, smudging with sage or other herbs, or using crystals or other energy-clearing tools. The intention is to remove any energy blockages and promote the free flow of positive energy throughout the body.

Both shielding and clearing energy practices can promote well-being and maintain a positive energy balance.

There are many ways to practice energy shielding, and what works best for one person may not work for another. Here are a few examples of energy shielding techniques:

1. *Visualize a protective shield*: One of the simplest ways to create an energy shield is to visualize a protective barrier around yourself. This can be done by closing your eyes and imagining a bubble of white light surrounding you or visualizing a suit of armor or a shield made of protective material, such as gold or silver.
2. *Use crystals*: Certain crystals, such as black tourmaline or obsidian, are believed to be particularly effective at blocking negative energy. Carrying or wearing these crystals or placing them in your home or workspace can help to create a protective energy shield.
3. *Use protective symbols*: Symbols or crystals with protective properties can help us shield.
4. *Call on our higher self, spiritual guides, or angels*: You can simply ask for their help or visualize them surrounding you with their protective energy.
5. *Ground yourself*: Walking barefoot in nature or visualizing yourself rooted in the earth can help to create a sense of stability and protection. This can help to prevent negative energy from entering your energy field in the first place.

Remember, finding a technique that resonates with you and feels adequate for your needs is the most important thing.

MY PERSONAL RECOMMENDATIONS AND SUGGESTIONS

Building a shield can also be done with the help of a trusted practitioner. Understanding your ability to hold this shield before working in the higher dimensional realms is important. I can help with clearing attachments/tech and shielding if you need support.

Here are my recommendations for energy shielding to get started:

1. Listen to the higher self-meditation, and journey back there with calming music a few times.

   https://youtu.be/Vo9vGFbzYEg

2. Create a really good connection to your higher self.
3. You can then create your own sacred space or use the space with the tree in my meditation and make it your own.
4. Create a shield that feels comfortable. The shape will be something unique to you.
5. Connect with your shield often initially and understand its energy and how it protects and works with you. It is a sentient being that is just there to lean on for anything needed. Sometimes, it locks me in super tight, and sometimes it is just a free-flowing feeling around me. Ensure you ground your energy back into your body when you come back down.
6. Build the shield and see how it feels.
7. Clearing, protection, and recalibration can be checked on daily as a good hygiene practice.

Example of what I do daily:

1. Every night, I clear energy from the day and look at my family. I just run a scan down my body and shield and ask to see if anything around it needs to be removed. There shouldn't be anything getting through the shield, but sometimes you may feel things around the shield affecting your energy.

It becomes a super fast scan, and I don't even notice my shield unless it is needed to add support. Initially, I asked to see all the tech, dark energy, density, and anything around my shield, self, house, or family.

Decree that can be said to clear energy.

- I do not consent to any form of tech, negative energy, or manipulation that will feed on my weaknesses and undermine my authority to be sovereign and in my personal power.
- I do not consent to any form of negative interference with my energy. I am supported by and connected to pure higher dimensional frequencies, and all impurities are continuously cleared and removed, whether from conscious or unconscious agreement and understanding.
- I am supported and protected by my internal guidance and higher self-connection. I go through the channel of my soul signature to receive messages or guidance, ensuring I am keeping my channel clear and clean.
- I return to my centered state of existence with grace and ease whenever I feel unbalanced, or my energy is low.
- Upgrades can be adjusted to fit my speed of integration at any time by simply checking in with my body and what is needed.
- I replace all that no longer serves my highest good with the best intentions for growth and prosperity in all timelines across all planes of reality.

CHAPTER 10

ENERGY WORK TO HELP THE HEALING JOURNEY

I cannot express this enough: <u>energy clearing and healing work led to an entirely different me.</u>

Energy work is holistic healing involving the body's subtle energy systems to promote balance, harmony, and well-being. The idea is that the body has an energetic or "vital" force that can be influenced and manipulated through various techniques.

Here are some examples of energy work:

1. *Quantum healing*: a form of energy healing that involves the practitioner channeling healing energy from higher dimensional frequencies; this can be hands-on or remote. The goal is to promote relaxation, reduce stress, and support the body's natural healing processes. This process can clear out density, which can speed up the process of healing and conscious expansion. (I work with this daily.)
2. *Acupuncture*: a form of Traditional Chinese Medicine that involves inserting fine needles into specific points on the body to stimulate the energy flow "qi." The goal of acupuncture is to restore balance and harmony to the body and promote healing. (this was key to stopping my migraines.
3. *Chakra balancing and healing*: Chakras are energy centers

in the body that are believed to correspond to different physical, emotional, and spiritual aspects of the self. Chakra balancing involves using various techniques, such as meditation, visualization, or energy work, to promote balance and harmony in the chakras. I did this a lot at the beginning of my journey, as it was easy to visualize. My favorite book when I started my healing practices was The Complete Book of Chakra Healing.

https://amzn.to/45Acy5R

4. *Auric fieldwork*: The auric field, also known as the aura, is an energy field that surrounds the body and is believed to contain information about our physical, emotional, and spiritual state. Auric fieldwork involves using various techniques, such as visualization, energy work, or sound healing, to clear and balance the aura. Promoting balance and harmony in the aura can support our health and well-being. (I work with this when clearing energy.)

5. *Akashic Records Healing*: I've worked in Akashic Records for years. Understanding my soul's history, what I am here to do, and working with others to heal and share messages has been a beautiful process. The records are known as the Book of Life and record the journey of our souls. Anyone can access their records by mediating and connecting in.

6. *Crystal healing*: Crystal healing involves using crystals and gemstones to balance and influence the body's energy systems. Different crystals are believed to have other properties and energies that can be used for healing and support. They have personalities and are very conscious. I love having them around and using them with my healing work.

7. *Sound healing*: Sound healing involves using sound vibrations, such as singing bowls, gongs, or tuning forks, to promote relaxation and balance in the body. The vibrations influence the body's energy systems and promote healing. My favorite sound healing is singing.

When a voice can bring me to tears, it hits that frequency unmatched by singing bowls or something of the sort.

8. *Past life healing*: Clearing, rewriting, and healing past life pain and suffering. Whew, this has been profound work. Understanding my past has made my present happier, my future goals more transparent, and allowed me to understand my mission. Why I am here and what I am here to do.

Energy work can be a powerful tool for promoting healing and well-being. Working with a qualified practitioner who can help guide you through the process and ensure that the techniques are safe and appropriate for your needs is important.

Depending on individual needs and goals, people may experience many benefits from working with the auric field and chakra balancing. Here are some common benefits that people may experience:

1. Reduced stress and anxiety: Alleviate anxiety by releasing tension and promoting greater harmony and balance in the body's energy systems.
2. Improved emotional well-being: Release emotional blockages and promote greater emotional stability and well-being.
3. Increased physical health: Support the body's natural healing processes, promote greater vitality, and alleviate physical symptoms.
4. Greater spiritual awareness: Promote greater spiritual awareness and connection by helping clear and open the energy centers in the body associated with spiritual growth and development.
5. Improved relationships: By promoting greater emotional well-being and spiritual awareness, enhancing relationships with ourselves and others is common.

CHAPTER 11

THE CHAKRA SYSTEM AND WOMB CONNECTION

Here are the seven main chakras, along with their associated colors, sounds, and functions:

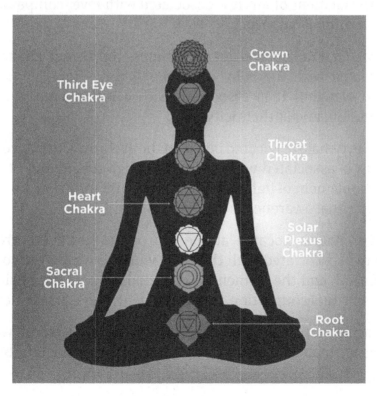

Root chakra: Located at the base of the spine, the root chakra is associated with the color red, the sound "Lam," and the element of earth. It is associated with grounding, stability, and survival.

Sacral chakra: Located just below the navel, the sacral chakra is associated with the color orange, the sound "Vam," and the water element. It is associated with creativity, pleasure, and sexuality.

Solar plexus chakra: Located above the navel, the solar plexus chakra is associated with the color yellow, the sound "Ram," and the fire element. It is related to personal power, self-esteem, and confidence.

Heart chakra: Located in the center of the chest, the heart chakra is associated with the color green, the sound "Yam," and the element of air. It is associated with love, compassion, and emotional balance.

Throat chakra: Located at the throat, the throat chakra is associated with the color blue, the sound "Ham," and the sound element. It is associated with communication, self-expression, and authenticity.

Third eye chakra: Located between the eyebrows, the third eye chakra is associated with the color indigo, the sound "Om," and the element of light. It is associated with intuition, insight, and spiritual awareness.

Crown chakra: Located at the top of the head, the crown chakra is associated with the color violet or white, the sound "Silence," and the element of consciousness. It is associated with spiritual connection, enlightenment, and transcendence.

Balancing and opening the chakras can promote overall well-being and maintain a healthy energy flow throughout the body.

SACRAL AND THROAT CONNECTION

The throat chakra is the first yoni, and the second yoni (or sacral chakra) are two of the seven main chakras in the body according to the Indian tradition of yoga.

The throat chakra is located in the throat area and is associated with communication, self-expression, creativity, and the ability to speak one's truth. When the throat chakra is balanced and open, you can communicate clearly and effectively, express yourself creatively, and feel confident speaking your truth.

The second yoni, also known as the sacral chakra, is located in the lower abdomen and is associated with creativity, sexuality, pleasure, and emotional balance. When the second yoni is balanced and open, an individual can experience pleasure and intimacy in a healthy and balanced way and express their creativity freely.

There is a connection between the throat and sacral, as both relate to the ability to express oneself and connect with others meaningfully. When the second yoni is blocked or imbalanced, it can lead to difficulty expressing oneself, low self-esteem, and difficulty forming intimate relationships. Similarly, when the throat chakra is blocked or imbalanced, it can lead to difficulty communicating effectively, feeling misunderstood, and a lack of confidence in one's ability to express oneself.

Working on balancing and opening these chakras through various practices, such as yoga, meditation, energy work, or therapy, can help to improve communication and self-expression, enhance creativity and sexuality, and promote emotional balance and well-being.

I also reference the importance of the Earth and Soul Star Chakras with the primary seven.

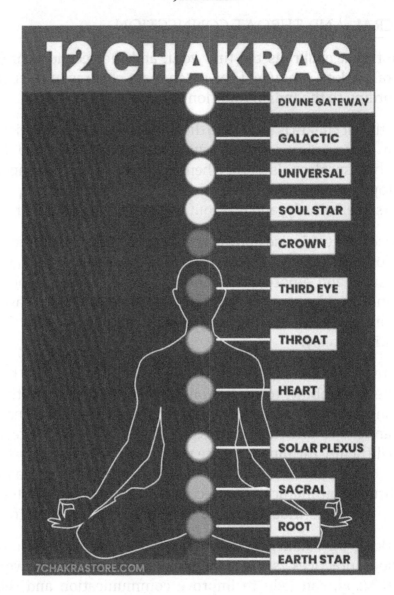

EARTH STAR CHAKRA

The Earth Star chakra is a relatively lesser-known chakra in the human energy system, located below the feet in the Earth's energy field.

The Earth Star chakra is associated with grounding, stability, and physical connection to the Earth. The chakra connects individuals to their ancestral roots, cultural heritage, and lineage. It is also believed to be the chakra that connects individuals to the collective consciousness of the Earth and the wisdom and knowledge of the natural world.

Several practices can help to balance and open the Earth Star chakra, including grounding exercises, meditation, spending time in nature, and connecting with one's cultural heritage and lineage. By working with the Earth Star chakra, individuals can deepen their connection to the Earth and their roots and gain a greater sense of stability and grounding in their lives.

SOUL STAR CHAKRA

The Soul Star chakra is associated with spiritual connection, higher consciousness, and the divine. The chakra connects individuals to their higher self, spiritual guides, and universal consciousness.

When the Soul Star chakra is balanced and open, an individual can access higher levels of consciousness, spiritual guidance, and a deeper understanding of their purpose and path in life. They may feel a stronger connection to the divine and greater peace and fulfillment.

Several practices can help to balance and open the Soul Star chakra, including meditation, energy work, connecting with spiritual guides, and exploring one's spiritual path and purpose. By working with the Soul Star chakra, individuals can deepen their spiritual connection and understanding and gain a greater sense of purpose and fulfillment in life. Placing your tongue on top/roof of your mouth activates the Soul Star and can help overall chakra alignment.

CHAPTER 12

CLAIR GIFTS AND PRACTICE

Clair gifts, psychic or intuitive gifts, are abilities that some people have to perceive information beyond what can be perceived through the five senses. There are several different types of Clair gifts, including:

Clairvoyance: This is the ability to see things not visible to the naked eye, such as images, symbols, or colors.

Clairaudience: This is the ability to hear things that are not audible to the ears, such as voices, music, or sounds.

Clairsentience: This is the ability to feel or sense things that are not tangible, such as emotions, energies, or physical sensations.

Claircognizance: This is the ability to know things without any apparent source of information or evidence.

Clairalience: This is the ability to smell things that are not present, such as scents or odors.

Clairgustance: This is the ability to taste things that are not present, such as flavors or substances.

Everyone has Clair gifts, and they may use them for a variety of purposes, such as spiritual guidance, healing, or intuitive counseling. It's important to note that these gifts are natural abilities that can be developed and honed over time.

If you are interested in exploring and opening your clair gifts with assistance, I can help. It's also important to approach these gifts with an open and grounded mindset and to use them in a way that is ethical, respectful, and compassionate toward others.

To strengthen your Clair gifts, working with your higher self and multidimensional aspects can help guide you and keep you moving to your best and highest potential and timeline.

Higher self: The higher self is the part of us connected to our spiritual essence or soul. It is often described as the part of us that is wise, compassionate, and connected to a higher power or universal consciousness. When we connect with our higher self, we can tap into a greater sense of purpose, meaning, and guidance.

Multidimensional aspects are aspects of us in higher dimensions, similar to spirit guides. They may also be versions of us in parallel realities. In addition to our physical body and the material world, we may also have energetic, emotional, mental, and spiritual aspects that exist on different levels of reality. We can promote greater wholeness, balance, and well-being by exploring and integrating these various aspects of ourselves.

MUSCLE TESTING

Muscle testing, also known as kinesiology, is a technique used to assess the strength or weakness of muscles in response to various stimuli. It is often used in alternative and complementary medicine practices to diagnose health issues, identify allergies or food sensitivities, and test the effectiveness of treatments.

During muscle testing, the practitioner applies pressure to a muscle while the patient resists the pressure. This can also be done individually. The muscle's response is then evaluated to determine its strength or weakness.

There are many examples in The Emotion Code and The Body Code books and online. The important thing is to make sure you have a good baseline so your ego is not interfering with the answers. These books are beneficial in understanding how to clear trapped emotions.

https://amzn.to/3SukRNM

https://amzn.to/3u21xNX

SWAY TEST

The sway test is muscle testing often used in alternative and complementary medicine practices to assess the body's response to various stimuli. It is sometimes called the "body sway method" or "body dowsing."

During the sway test, you stand upright with your feet shoulder-width apart and arms extended to the sides. Observe the body to see if it sways forward or backward in response to the stimulus. Forward can be yes, and back can be no.

PENDULUM

A pendulum is a weight attached to a string or chain to answer yes or no questions. The pendulum is often made of a crystal, metal, or wood and can be used for divination, energy healing, and other spiritual practices. Please clear and cleanse any tools before using them.

To use a pendulum, hold the end of the chain or string with their fingers and allow the weight to hang freely. Ask a yes or no question or pose a query and observe the pendulum's movement. The pendulum may swing back and forth in a circular motion or other patterns, depending on the answer to the question or the information being conveyed.

Many Clair gift exercises can be found online. I always say, "Practice, practice, practice!" as this will help you grow your gifts (it doesn't happen magically with no effort).

Some of my favorites are imagining an orange getting peeled or challenging yourself to see yes or no answers in your third eye.

Practicing hearing things outside the room, then moving out further and further to say the house, block, subdivision, town, state, world, etc.

Meditation can help to quiet the mind and develop your ability to focus and concentrate. This can help build your Clair abilities, as it requires a similar level of focus and concentration.

Keep a dream journal: Dreams can be a powerful way to tap into your Clair abilities, as they often contain symbolic messages or information beyond the physical realm. Keeping a dream journal and recording your dreams can help you better understand and develop your clairvoyant abilities.

Practice energy work: Working with energy can help to build your clairsentient abilities and increase your sensitivity to subtle energy.

READING ORACLE CARDS

Oracle and Tarot cards are divination tools often used for spiritual guidance, self-reflection, and personal growth. They typically feature images and symbols designed to convey specific messages or insights. I used Oracle cards to help me strengthen my connection and trust my intuition and the answers I received at the beginning of my healing work daily.

If you are interested in reading Oracle cards, here are some steps you can follow:

1. Choose a deck: There are many different types of Oracle card decks available, each with unique themes, symbols, and messages. Choose a deck that resonates with you and that you feel drawn to. Here are a few of my favorite decks.

   Sacred Forest

   https://amzn.to/3RvVpqy

   Dragon Oracle cards

   https://amzn.to/3RvViv8

   Earth Warriors

   https://amzn.to/44QwlOJ

   The Light Seer's Tarot

   https://amzn.to/3Znmbn5

   The Rider Tarot Deck

   https://amzn.to/3QA7tpX

   The Ultimate Guide to Tarot

   https://amzn.to/478MMa3

2. Set your intention: Before beginning a reading, it can be helpful to set your intention and ask for guidance from your higher self, spirit guides, or other spiritual allies.

3. Shuffle the cards: Shuffle the cards while focusing on your question or intention. You can shuffle the cards in any way that feels comfortable, such as by spreading them out on a table, mixing them around, or holding them in your hands and shuffling them like a regular deck. The decks may also have specific ways to read the cards.

4. Draw a card: Draw a card from the deck once ready. Take a

moment to look at the image and symbols on the card and see what messages or insights come to mind.

5. Reflect on the card's meaning: Each card in the deck will have its unique meaning and message, which your specific question or intention may influence. Reflect on the card's meaning and how it relates to your current situation or question.

6. Trust your intuition: When reading oracle cards, it is important to trust your intuition and allow your inner wisdom to guide you. Don't worry too much about following strict rules or interpretations - instead, let the cards speak to you in a way that feels authentic and meaningful.

CHAPTER 13

SEXUAL HEALING

The concept of "womb sexual healing", is a term that can have different meanings to different people. However, generally speaking, it refers to healing any emotional, physical, or energetic imbalances in the reproductive system that may affect a person's sexual health and well-being. I had trouble feeling comfortable with my body due to the childhood abuse. There were times I felt like I was completely numb when doing this work. There was physical pain, nausea, emotion, and not even wanting to be touched by my husband. Things that come up are natural and normal, and it is essential to communicate with a spouse or partner as you do this work so they can understand and help support your process.

There are many different approaches to womb sexual healing, and what works for one person may not work for another. Our sexual energy is sacred, and we should honor our wombs and our bodies. Many manifestation practices go into using the sexual energy to get what we want faster. I do not recommend this, as it opens up a gateway to things we do not want to connect with.

It is also important to understand the higher frequency individual takes on the energy of the lower individual during intercourse. As you heal, you may realize who you are attracted to and want to be around changes. Check-in with your higher self to ensure your significant other is an energetic match when in the dating pool.

Distorted sexual energy is vital to understand.

Distorted sexual energy can manifest in various ways. Here are a few potential indicators that may suggest the presence of distorted sexual energy:

Obsessive or compulsive sexual thoughts: If someone is constantly preoccupied with sexual thoughts or experiences an overwhelming urge to engage in sexual activities that disrupt their daily life and functioning, it may be a sign of distorted sexual energy.

Self-destructive sexual behaviors: Engaging in risky or harmful sexual behaviors, such as unprotected sex, promiscuity, or engaging in sexual activities that cause physical or emotional harm, can be indicative of distorted sexual energy.

Lack of boundaries and consent: Disregarding personal boundaries or the boundaries of others or engaging in non-consensual sexual activities is a significant red flag. Healthy sexual energy respects consent and establishes clear boundaries.

Guilt, shame, or secrecy: Feeling intense guilt or shame surrounding one's sexuality or sexual desires can indicate distorted sexual energy.

Emotional detachment or avoidance: If someone consistently uses sex to avoid emotional intimacy or numb themselves from emotional pain, it could be a sign of distorted sexual energy. Healthy sexual energy embraces both physical and emotional connection.

Inability to form healthy relationships: Struggling to establish and maintain healthy, fulfilling relationships may indicate distorted sexual energy. This can manifest as difficulties with trust, intimacy, or forming deeper emotional connections.

Sexual addiction: When an individual cannot control their sexual urges and engages in compulsive or excessive sexual behaviors that may negatively impact their personal relationships, work, or overall well-being.

Pornography addiction: Excessive consumption of pornography can distort one's perception of healthy sexuality, leading to unrealistic expectations, objectification of others, and difficulties forming healthy intimate relationships.

Sexual shame and guilt: Cultural or religious beliefs, societal norms, or personal experiences can contribute to feelings of shame or guilt surrounding one's sexual desires or behaviors. This can lead to a distorted view of sexuality and hinder healthy sexual expression.

Approach these signs with compassion and understanding but also understand warning signs as underlying issues could be coming to the surface to heal or showing up as red flags when picking partners.

CHAPTER 14

THE HEAVY LIFTING AND DEEPER TRAUMA CLEARING

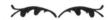

I have seen some severe trauma cause loops and trouble moving through things. In these cases, the healing may take longer. This is not the same thing as deeper layers of trauma clearing but reliving events without releasing the stored trauma, similar to PTSD. These instances will most likely need longer assistance. Not to be confused with resistance to doing the work and avoiding the work. This is where our safety center can not pull us out of the depths of the trauma. So, we are constantly in the loop, feeling unsafe and unable to move forward.

However, this work can be fast-moving, and I am honest about timeframes when I work with people. I work directly with your higher self and the information most needed for your journey, not necessarily about speed but about integration at the greatest degree and tools to help along the way. I absolutely love watching the big shifts in people.

Trying to rush integration can be counterproductive. There needs to be time for the healing to settle in. My most incredible mentors were honest with love and compassion. I am forever grateful for this method as it moved even the most stuck energy as quickly and efficiently as possible without compounding layers I wasn't ready to process yet.

I highly recommend asking for help and guidance to move trauma, heal your womb, and have a space holder to support you with what needs to be integrated.

DNA AND RNA HEALING CRYSTALLINE UPGRADING, SEAL REMOVAL

DNA healing is a term that refers to various energy healing practices that aim to activate or unlock the full potential of the DNA within the cells of the body. Our DNA contains not only our genetic material but also our spiritual and energetic potential, and unlocking this potential can lead to profound healing and transformation on physical, emotional, and spiritual levels. I found DNA healing early on in my journey.

Diet, meditation, affirmations, sound healing, and connecting with your body can help you reach your full potential by unlocking your DNA and Crystalline blueprint.

Your DNA is sacred as it connects to your multidimensional experiences. Working with your higher self can repair and activate the etheric DNA strands. This process should happen naturally, but many years ago, we experienced a fall on the Earth plane, and this fall created issues and allowed seals or energetic fences to alter and halt DNA and Earth's ascension. This has been part of the reason we are experiencing progressive and degenerative issues. It is a very exciting time as we naturally return to our original blueprint.

When DNA is activated, it brings healing and a deeper connection. People have experienced relief from physical and emotional issues, especially anxiety. The natural progression is stopped at the 4th strand. This is where emotions can back up, or unexplained problems can suddenly occur.

We can open up to our natural gifts and hidden codes as we enter the Golden Age more efficiently than ever before. We all came down here with light codes. These codes help show purpose and bring you closer to joy and peace.

Below is a graph of some seals or energetic fences that can be cleared. There are more advanced things like Archon tech and implants, But these are the basics. As we evolve, some of these pop off naturally.

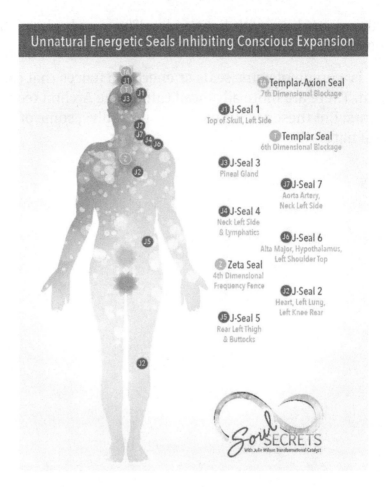

J Seals – These seals were placed on Earth's Grid years ago. The primary purpose is to keep us from being able to ascend. They cause progressive deterioration of the physical body. They mainly affect the left side of the body and the energetic circulatory system of the body.

J-1 (Left, Skull)

J-2 (Alta Major, Hypothalamus, Left Shoulder Top)

J-3 (Pineal Gland) This was removed years ago

J-4 (neck, lymphatic system)

J-5 (rear L thigh, buttocks)

J-6 (alta major: the way the skull rests on the spine, hypothalamus, left shoulder),

J-7 (aorta artery on L side of neck)

Zeta Seal – This seal affects our ability to evolve towards unconditional love and access to higher dimensions. It's an energetic "fence" blocking us spiritually from remembering our dreams, out-of-body experiences, and lucid dreams. It also blocks our intuitive gifts.

Death Seal – Everyone has a Death Seal; they were placed on the DNA so we as humans would live short lives, and it also kept us reincarnating repeatedly. This seal is a genetic seal handed down through hereditary lines.

Crown of Thorns – This seal was placed on our DNA to block and distort the natural energetic circulatory system, block our connection to our Higher Selves, and scramble the universal currents in the Chakras. (When this is removed, you might experience a taste of metal in your mouth).

Templar Seal | Templar-Axion Seal – The Templar seal is located in the center of the forehead, covering the 3rd eye. The Templar Axion seal is also known as the 666 seal. It affects the tones of the DNA strands 1, 5, and 6. The Templar Axion seal causes one to be buried in religious judgment, i.e., fear of the wrath of God or disbelief in a Higher Power whatsoever.

Seal of Amenti – The seal of Amenti was placed on the DNA willingly by all the members of the order of Isis and anyone who inappropriately shared sacred information from the Halls of Amenti as retribution for their infraction. It directly affects the Lymphatic system and the blood.

The Gene Keys book by Richard Rudd is helpful for shadow work and expansion. When I studied DNA healing, I also spent time on the Gene Key graphs and understanding how we can get stuck in cycles and loops. Each key represents a shadow, a gift, and a siddhi. Your role is to become aware of the shadow and how it shows up so that you can acknowledge and embrace that shadow part of you until it transmutes into the gift and siddhi.

SOUL FRAGMENT RETRIEVAL AND PAST LIFE HEALING

Soul fragment retrieval is a spiritual practice that involves identifying and reintegrating parts of the soul that have become disconnected or fragmented due to trauma, loss, or other life experiences. When we experience trauma, a part of our soul may become separated or disconnected to protect ourselves from further harm.

When this happens, we may experience symptoms such as feeling disconnected from ourselves or others, lost or ungrounded, or experiencing chronic physical or emotional pain. Soul fragment retrieval involves identifying these disconnected parts of the soul and working to reintegrate them back into the whole.

There are various ways to retrieve these aspects and parts of ourselves, such as shamanic journeying, guided meditation, or energy healing. Practitioners may use techniques such as visualization, intention-setting, or energy work to help identify and retrieve these fragmented parts of the soul.

Similarly, past life healing can bring up intense emotions. When we start meditating, we often get specific memories that come in but are only part of the picture. When I was first learning how to read the Akashic records, I had past lives come in to heal and didn't understand the whole scene until I was ready to go that deep. I think of it as doing a puzzle; we get sections we are prepared for, and the entire puzzle is put together when we are ready to integrate the information. If we keep asking for what is next, the answers or the person needed to help us gain clarity appears at some point. Sometimes, this can take days, months, and years to understand. Keeping notes or a journal is helpful so you can go back to things when more comes in.

I almost always work with past and parallel life healing and soul fragment retrieval in my client sessions. Sometimes, birthmarks, fears, and phobias are linked to past events. Many fears of heights, water, certain animals, etc., can be cleared through this work. This is also where we find the answers as to why we are drawn to or repelled by certain people, places, or things.

Working with an experienced practitioner who can guide you through the process and provide support and guidance can be helpful, especially for the first few times you do it.

SUPPRESSED MEMORY RETRIEVAL

Repressed memories are memories blocked from conscious awareness due to trauma or other intense emotional experiences. This is why I had chunks of time completely gone from childhood.

Several methods have been used to retrieve repressed memories, including hypnosis, guided imagery, and other forms of healing. I never reacted to hypnosis. I tried a couple of times. But it was always just blank, with me questioning what I was supposed to say.

It is also extremely important you know how to process emotion. This work should be done with the help of a safe and supportive environment so that you have guidance and support as you work through any trauma or emotional experiences that may have contributed to repressing your memories.

Many times, sexual abuse from childhood can come up with this work. When the memories are retrieved, they can cause emotion, depression, physical nausea, and pain in your stomach, heart, and womb. You will also need a solid foundation of understanding shadow work and how to move through deeper trauma. This takes trusting yourself and the information that comes through, as the first thing that usually happens is denial and wanting to repress what's challenging to feel.

I was alone for most of the processing when I found my memories. Someone needs to hold the space so that you can process and feel supported instead of feeling that you have to do it on your own or alone. This doesn't mean you have to relive every single event, but understanding what happened and how to heal what is left in your body is important.

ANCESTRAL HEALING

Another type of beneficial healing is ancestral healing. Ancestral healing is a type of healing that focuses on addressing and releasing ancestral trauma, patterns, and wounds that may be affecting individuals in the present.

Ancestral healing can involve various practices, including meditation, visualization, energy healing, and family constellations. These practices aim to identify and heal ancestral wounds, patterns, and beliefs that may affect an individual's physical, emotional, and spiritual well-being.

Ancestral healing can be a powerful and transformative process. Mediumship often comes through in my healing sessions as loved ones who have passed want to share messages with us. So, this can be a beautiful way to heal the family ties. I cleared the lineage of the abuse in my childhood once I healed enough.

ENERGY CONTRACT CLEARING

Energy contract clearing is a type of energy healing practice that involves identifying and releasing energetic contracts or agreements that may affect an individual's well-being. These contracts may be conscious or unconscious and may be created with other people, organizations, or spiritual entities.

Energy contract clearing aims to identify and release any contracts or agreements that no longer serve an individual's highest good and create space for new and positive energies to enter. This can involve identifying any limiting beliefs or patterns connected to the contracts and working to release them through various energy-healing modalities, chakra balancing, or guided visualization.

One common practice in energy contract clearing is to work with a qualified energy healer or Akashic records practitioner who can help identify and release any energetic contracts or agreements that may affect an individual's well-being. Contracts, vows, and curses can all come up when diving into contract clearing. It can be a short, simple process or go deep into layers of healing the lineage. This may involve a combination of energy healing techniques and guidance on setting healthy boundaries and creating positive, energetic relationships moving forward.

It is important to approach energy contract clearing with an open mind and to work with a qualified practitioner with years of experience in this area.

SUBCONSCIOUS LIMITING BELIEFS CLEARING

Subconscious limiting belief clearing is a type of personal development practice that involves identifying and releasing limiting beliefs that may be holding an individual back from reaching their full potential. These beliefs are often deeply ingrained in the subconscious mind and may be formed in childhood or early life experiences, cultural conditioning, or other factors.

The goal of subconscious limiting beliefs is to identify and transform them, replacing them with more positive and empowering beliefs supporting an individual's growth and success.

One common practice in subconscious limiting belief clearing is to use affirmations or positive statements to reprogram the subconscious mind. This may involve repeating positive affirmations or visualizations that reinforce positive beliefs and help to release limiting beliefs.

It is important to approach subconscious limiting beliefs clearing with patience and self-compassion, as this process can take time and may involve exploring deep-seated emotions and beliefs. I can also help with this work if you feel stuck or if a particular belief keeps recycling.

Remember, the beliefs we hold about ourselves and the world around us can have a profound impact on our lives. By identifying and releasing limiting beliefs, we can create space for positive change and growth and cultivate a greater sense of self-awareness and empowerment.

The goal of subconscious limiting beliefs clearing is to bring these beliefs to the conscious level, identify their roots, and release them. By releasing these limiting beliefs, individuals can create new positive beliefs and patterns that support their personal growth and success.

Another approach is to use self-help tools, such as journaling, meditation, or visualization, to identify and release limiting beliefs. These techniques can help individuals become more aware of their negative self-talk and patterns and develop strategies for replacing them with positive beliefs and affirmations.

I do a simple visualization with my daughter each night before bed, where we clear out anything from the day and replace it with beautiful animals and happy energies.

CHAPTER 15
CONNECTING WITH THE DIVINE FEMININE

WAYS TO EXPLORE THE DIVINE FEMININE

The archetype of the Divine Feminine is a concept that has been present in many cultures and spiritual traditions throughout history. It represents the feminine aspects of the divine, including nurturing, compassion, intuition, creativity, and wisdom. Exploring this archetype can be a powerful way to connect with our inner wisdom and feminine power.

Connect with nature: Spending time in nature, especially in natural settings such as forests, oceans, or rivers, can help us connect with the nurturing and creative power of the Divine Feminine. Take time to observe the natural world and notice the cycles of birth, growth, and transformation.

Practice self-care: The Divine Feminine is associated with nurturing and self-care. Taking time to care for ourselves, whether through taking a bath, practicing yoga, or spending time with loved ones, can help us connect with our nurturing power.

Access intuition: The Divine Feminine is associated with intuition and inner wisdom. Journaling, meditation, or divination can help us access this inner wisdom and connect with our intuition.

Embrace creativity: The Divine Feminine is associated with creativity and the arts. Engaging in creative practices such as painting, writing, singing, or dance can help us connect with our creative power and express ourselves in new ways.

Remember, exploring the archetype of the Divine Feminine can be a powerful tool for connecting with our inner wisdom and feminine power. It's important to approach the process with patience and self-compassion and to allow ourselves to explore and discover what resonates with us.

CEREMONIES TO HONOR THE WOMB

Here are a few examples of ceremonies that can be incorporated into a womb-healing practice:

Setting Sacred Space: Begin by creating a sacred space where you feel safe and comfortable. This can be a quiet room, a natural outdoor setting, or any place to connect with your inner self.

Meditation and Breathwork: Start the ritual with a meditation or breathwork practice. Close your eyes, focus on your breath, and visualize healing energy flowing into your womb space. You can use affirmations or mantras that resonate with you, such as "I am worthy of healing" or "I embrace my feminine power."

Sacred Bath: Take a ceremonial bath infused with herbs or essential oils known for their healing properties. You can add herbs like rose petals, lavender, chamomile, or yarrow to the bathwater. As you soak, visualize the healing energy penetrating your womb space and releasing any stagnant or negative energy.

Womb Massage: Perform a gentle womb massage using warm oils such as sweet almond, jojoba, or rosehip. Use circular motions on your lower abdomen, connecting with your womb. This massage can help increase blood flow, release tension, and promote energetic balance.

Affirmations and Mantras: Repeat positive affirmations and mantras specific to womb healing. Affirmations such as "My womb is a sacred space of creativity and power" or "I release any past traumas and embrace my divine feminine energy" can be empowering and supportive.

Remember, these ceremonies are meant to be personalized and adapted to your own beliefs and needs. Trust your intuition and create a practice that resonates with you. It may also be beneficial to seek guidance from experienced practitioners or explore teachings from various traditions specializing in womb healing.

CULTIVATING A RELATIONSHIP WITH THE DIVINE FEMININE FOR WOMB HEALING

Cultivating a relationship with the Divine Feminine can be a powerful tool for womb healing. Here are some practices that can help you connect with the Divine Feminine and cultivate a deeper relationship for womb healing:

1. *Honoring your womb*: One way to connect with the Divine Feminine for womb healing is to honor your womb as a sacred space. You can create a special altar or space in your home dedicated to your womb and the Divine Feminine. You can also practice self-care rituals such as taking a warm bath, using essential oils, or doing gentle yoga poses that support your womb.

2. *Connecting with nature*: Spending time in nature can help you connect with the Divine Feminine and the earth's natural cycles. You can walk in the woods, spend time by the ocean, or simply sit outside and connect with the earth's energy.

3. *Working with crystals*: Crystals can be a powerful tool for womb healing and connecting with the Divine Feminine. You can work with crystals such as moonstone, rose quartz, or carnelian, which are associated with the womb

and feminine energy. I like to hold crystals while I meditate or put them on my chakra centers.

4. *Journaling*: Journaling can be a powerful tool for connecting with your inner wisdom and the Divine Feminine. You can use journaling prompts such as "What does my womb need to heal?" or "What messages does the Divine Feminine have for me?" to explore your inner world and connect with your intuition.

5. *Meditation*: Meditations can be a powerful tool for connecting with the Divine Feminine and accessing your inner wisdom. You can find guided meditations online or through apps, or work with a teacher or healer specializing in guided meditations for womb healing.

6. *Oracle Decks*: Working with Oracle decks of Divine Feminine energies. 2018, I used the Goddess Guidance Oracle Cards by Doreen Virtue, but it is out of print and overpriced now.

Goddess Power by Collette Baron Reid is a good replacement.

https://amzn.to/3EEEpqE

Keepers of the Light by Kyle Gray.

https://amzn.to/48jWnMQ

Many times, I would just connect in meditation, and a guide would come to me, and I would find out who she was after if her image wasn't clear. I mainly meditated with my higher self when connecting with goddess energy.

You can work with feminine energies like Mary Magdelene for positive feminine energy. For darker feminine energy goddess types, I only ever worked with Hekate and Persephone, as both were there to help me balance the lower frequencies and understand how to bounce back and forth. I don't recommend working with darker female archetypes until you can discern their history. Not everything written necessarily paints the entire picture of history. Self-love and understanding that all parts of you can shine are essential when doing this work. Let the goddess who wants to work with you present herself. What happened in the past is over.

Allow yourself to explore different practices and find what resonates with you.

DIVINE UNION

Once you work with your Divine Feminine energy, if you are drawn to embody and find your inner and outer Divine Union, Acacia Lawson can guide you through this process. She is my go-to for Divine Union work.

https://www.facebook.com/acacia.lawson.3

Divine Union is a spiritual concept that refers to the merging of the masculine and feminine energies within a person and the resulting sense of wholeness and balance. It is often associated with finding one's soulmate and is seen as a symbol of spiritual completion and fulfillment.

In many spiritual traditions, a divine union is associated with the concept of the divine masculine and divine feminine, which are seen as complementary energies that exist within all human beings. These energies are believed to represent different aspects of the divine, such as strength, power, and action (masculine), and love, compassion, and intuition (feminine).

Achieving divine union involves integrating these energies within oneself and balancing them to create a sense of inner harmony and wholeness. This happens after healing trauma, past lives, the womb, etc., and includes meditation, energy work, and other spiritual practices that help awaken and balance these inner energies.

In the context of relationships, divine union is often seen as the ultimate goal of a romantic partnership, where both individuals can merge their energies in a way that creates a deep sense of connection, love, and mutual support that goes beyond the physical reality.

Overall, divine union emphasizes the importance of balance and integration in all aspects of life, including spiritual, emotional, and relational. By achieving a state of inner harmony and balance, individuals can experience a greater sense of fulfillment, purpose, and connection to the divine.

CHAPTER 16

CONCLUSION

I think that about sums up what got me here—a little of everything from beginning to end. I started my healing journey because my body was shutting down. I wanted my daughter to have a happy childhood. I was concerned that history would repeat itself and wanted to clear everything connected to my childhood assault. I held pain for so long that wasn't mine to carry and only learned how to unpack it as an adult. My happiness and joy are a direct result of my work. I healed my body and continue to work on any density/trauma that comes up when it is ready to be released, and my body just gets stronger every day. It is a spiral; we just keep going and connecting deeper to who we are. Everything that happens to us makes us stronger, not weaker, and we have so much potential. I feel like my process could have taken less time had I known all the things I know now.

But there is another huge reason I wanted to share this book. It stems from something that happened a couple of years ago and has stayed with me since.

We are incredibly sentimental in my house. My daughter always wants to surprise us with something. So she had my husband help her order a <u>What I love about Mom </u>book. At age 8, she wrote 1-50 things in this book, and the theme was about my healing work from her perspective of what that meant. I always shared how to work with energy, clearing, and meditation. Obviously, the heavier work was not shared. However, there were moments she would see me cry while processing and hug me. I always made sure to let her know emotions are not bad and that sometimes we cry not because we are mad at someone but just because it's how the energy shifts out the old that needs to go. She loves crystals, so we always talked about chakras and where they were in the body and put crystals on them when she would ask to mediate with me. She has always been curious, and I love that she is interested. I cried the day I read that book. It was the best acknowledgment for this journey I could have gotten.

There were several references to healing in those 50 things. My daughter loved the adventures we took in meditation. She loved how she felt when I did energy work on her. The rest of that book was about how she loved homeschooling (this was forced at first when all the children were sent home and a blessing in the fact I couldn't imagine doing it a different way now).

She went on to talk about her love for our connection, her dogs, and spending time together laughing and listening to music. She emphasized how I let her feel her feelings no matter what they were and that she could always talk to me about anything.

While I have definitely made mistakes along the way, each layer has left me feeling lighter, happier, and more equipped to be the best version of myself possible. The person I was when I first started healing is a distant memory. Even my pictures and videos back then look like a different me.

And this is why the heavy lifting is important, to clear this energy from ourselves, for our kids and our families, as well as for our communities and our world - and this is why this workbook came to life. The next generation is watching and taking notes. But more than anything, joy and happiness are our birthright.

My hope is that we change the world together, one step at a time! I am sending you so much love and healing on your journey. Please reach out to me if you have any questions or need any further guidance!

Julie

P.S. Once you complete this workbook, email me at healingwithjw@gmail.com to get a certificate of completion.

If you received help from this book, please take a moment to leave an Amazon review. It really helps self-published authors to make a bigger impact. Thank you!

RESOURCES

Also on QR Code
Pictures of exercises from Pinterest various sites

https://www.youtube.com/channel/
UClzZuzFm0wFEcUXgx6Nsigg

https://www.youtube.com/watch?v=dKBEqL4PZvQ

https://www.youtube.com/watch?v=L1HCG3BGK8I&t=2s

https://www.youtube.com/watch?v=XFFDWwQgIRM

https://www.youtube.com/watch?v=pAclBdj20ZU

https://www.youtube.com/watch?v=pAclBdj20ZU

https://youtu.be/hw8UjuXDcFU

https://www.youtube.com/watch?v=7JScerGmWrw&t=6s

https://youtu.be/FDuDgCZyGUg

https://youtu.be/2TePAocURL

My certifications and training

Acacia Lawson for Divine Union work

https://www.facebook.com/acacia.lawson.3

Youtube videos Eckart Tolle

YouTube videos Matt Khan

https://youtu.be/y2RAEnWreoE

Light of God Protocol *https://www.facebook.com/MTVOTeam/posts/2587305374815798*

https://youtube.com/shorts/ivToyrWC9bs?feature=share

https://secondnaturehealing.com/pineal-gland-spiritual-enlightenment/

https://www.gaia.com/article/pineal-third-eye-chakra

ABOUT THE AUTHOR

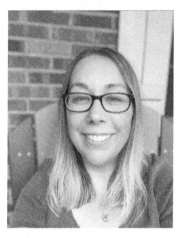

Julie Wilson is a multidimensional energy healer and facilitator. She has a close relationship with the energy of the Sacred Rose Order, Dragon energy, and many galactic councils. The early part of her journey was spent working through her healing process. She is creating a quantum healing method to help the integration of light codes while honoring individual sovereignty. Part of her mission is to protect innocence, honor children and their spiritual gifts, and help others step into their power.

Some of her specialties include helping people identify and expand spiritual gifts, tap into galactic history, past life healing, timeline work, DNA repair, mediumship, and supporting others through their healing journey. She also works with inner child and womb healing.

She is a homeschooling mom to a ten-year-old daughter, a wife, and a dog mom of two pups. She likes to travel, especially to the ocean, and spend time in nature. She loves being a mom because she is a kid at heart, and her husband never ceases to bring all the laughs (what we talk about as a prerequisite for marriage in this house). wink wink

If you would like to work with Julie, the link to her website is here, and don't hesitate to connect with her on Facebook.

Linktree:

https://linktr.ee/juliewilson111

Made in the USA
Monee, IL
09 October 2024

67531030R00089